The Colour of Madness

A groundbreaking collection edited by
Dr Samara Linton and Rianna Walcott

The Colour of Madness

Mental Health and Race in Technicolour

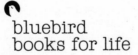
bluebird
books for life

This edition published 2022 by Bluebird
an imprint of Pan Macmillan
The Smithson, 6 Briset Street, London EC1M 5NR
EU representative: Macmillan Publishers Ireland Ltd, 1st Floor,
The Liffey Trust Centre, 117–126 Sheriff Street Upper,
Dublin 1, D01 YC43
Associated companies throughout the world
www.panmacmillan.com

ISBN 978-1-5290-8849-6

Typeset in Bell MT Std by Jouve (UK), Milton Keynes
Printed and bound by CPI Group (UK) Ltd, Croydon, CR0 4YY

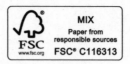

CONTENT WARNING

Many of the contributors talk about challenging experiences in their lives. Some readers might find the content of some of these accounts triggering, so we have added a symbol to the more detailed accounts to allow anyone who may find reading about sensitive content difficult the opportunity to pause.

For those past and present who were not able to tell their stories. For those who told their stories but were not heard. For those who are steeling themselves, waiting for their moment to speak.

Contents

Green

Polychrome

Artists' Notes

Blue

Indigo

Violet

'The most important voices to influence the improvement of our mental health services are those that live the experience of mental health challenges. The "Patient and Carer Race Equality Framework (PCREF)" enables service users, carers and community members to be involved in the re-imagination of services to respond to our needs in ways which are anti-racist, anti-discriminatory and anti-oppressive and support us to flourish. This book, which shares the poignant lived voices of the racialised experience, is a welcome contribution to that endeavour. We can draw strength from our stories and know that we are not alone in our struggles as we face relentless systemic racism. Indeed the sharing of our stories is purposeful in the mission to heal and positively transform our mental health, physical health and wellbeing.'

Dr Jacqui Dyer, Lived Expert by Experience,
Chair Advancing Mental Health Equalities Taskforce
and PCREF Steering Group (NHSEI),
Black Thrive Global Director

Editor's Introduction

Rianna Walcott

To our new readers, welcome, we are so glad to have you here! And to our returnees, welcome back, and thank you for your continued support.

Writing this again is bittersweet. Bitter, because the circumstances surrounding the recall of the original text are less than pleasant, and, in fact, reflect the worst of a struggle with white supremacy and the exploitation of people of colour that is endemic to the United Kingdom. Sweet, because it is a privilege to have the opportunity to give the collection new life in a moment when it is so dearly needed.

This isn't a revision in the exact sense of the word – we didn't get it wrong the first time around, and that edition remains one of our proudest accomplishments. Instead, we consider this a refinement. We have offered our contributors the opportunity to revise their contributions, to add to them, to reflect with postscripts, because the past four years have wrought changes that we could not have imagined when we first conceptualised *The Colour of Madness*.

A second chance

First, to address the elephant in the room. You may be aware already that this opportunity to republish comes at a heavy cost. The first edition was originally published in September 2018, and by March 2021 we had recovered the publishing rights. That first edition was a passion project, supported by an apparently benevolent and well-meaning indie publisher, Stirling Publishing Limited. Being passionate and optimistic twenty-three-year-olds who were new to the industry, Samara and I leapt at the opportunity that publishing director Tabatha Stirling presented, and brought together fifty-eight incredible artists, writers, and poets in the original collection. Looking back, I remain proud of all of us for the honesty, courage, and love that was poured into that first edition, and only regret that we did not understand our own power and value, or recognise the warning signs of a publisher who did not really know what they were doing.

Stirling Publishing Limited did not invest in marketing, press, or a book launch — we were even informed on the day of the launch that there were no copies of the book available. Based on these experiences we knew our publisher was incompetent, but at that time we thought it was their only sin, and Samara and I were nothing but efficient, picking up the slack. Still, we countered this incompetence with fierce determination, because this book was **good**; it was **necessary**; it was **worth it**.

We never dreamed that behind this lack of support something more sinister was lurking.

Finding out that our publisher was 'allegedly' a white supremacist was a blow. The news came to us from a Glasgow-based anti-fascist group, who had infiltrated the white ethno-nationalist group 'Patriotic Alternative' and found who they presumed to be our publisher writing hateful propaganda under the pseudonym Miss Britannia. They sought us out, asking for a positive identification. Given our extensive communication with Tabatha, I knew from the first few seconds of her tearful voice in a leaked WhatsApp voice note that it was her. She went on to identify

Stirling Publishing by name, as well as *The Colour of Madness*, dismissing us as a trendy way to make money, regretting publishing our beautiful book, claiming she had only sought us out because we were her ticket to BAME book awards.

Beyond the natural hurt and disgust that came with hearing her tearfully denounce people of multiple ethnicities, religions, and LGBTQ status, we were overcome by fear. Fear that her actions would taint the work, that the edition that she had almost ruined by her incompetence as a publisher would finally be killed in the cradle by her incompetence as a secret white supremacist.

Above all, we were horrified that this could impact our dear contributors, who had put their faith in us to find them a safe place for their stories. We were so vulnerable following this news, and it sickly paralleled the very vulnerability that the book was born out of – the struggle of existing and caring for your wellbeing in a country where white supremacy can fester under its skin.

And yet – here we are, again, back and better than ever! Thanks to the kindness and generosity of countless good people we were able to turn tragedy into success, reverting the rights to their work back to our contributors, and signing with Bluebird publishing. We lost some of our contributors along the way who, having made themselves vulnerable in print – some for the first time – were naturally wary of being betrayed a second time, but for the most part we are able to present you with the revised work of most of those original creators, and also have the privilege of including some new voices.

The continued importance of our stories being told by us, for us

This incident, to us, only reinforced the need for an outlet for our stories, and the importance of having control over the ways they were told. Part of that commitment led us to our change in subtitle, which was initially 'exploring BAME mental health in the UK', and is now 'race and mental health in technicolour'. The reason for the change is that we wanted to reflect something beyond the limitations of 'Black, Asian, and Minority Ethnic' (BAME), and we didn't want to prescribe how our contributors define themselves.

The value and beauty of this book is in its specificity, the fact that we are able to define our own experiences in and on our own terms. There is not always an overlap between those experiences, besides the shared narrative of being systemically disprivileged by the UK healthcare system. By using the more general umbrella of 'race', we invite our contributors to share the specifics with you in the way of their choosing. We also acknowledge the challenges around the term 'BAME', and the evolving conversation around self-definition as racialised people in this country.

We would be remiss to not mention the impact of the Covid-19 pandemic on the nation's health collectively, but also the specific impact it has had on racialised communities, in terms of both physical and mental health. The isolation of multiple lockdowns, disruption of communities and their networks of support, and the demonisation of people of colour globally as carriers of the virus would be bad enough. But the prevailing narrative of non-white communities in the UK as vaccine-hesitant and disinformation-rife, with little regard for histories of medical racism that contribute to this hesitancy, is still doing damage.

The public conversation around mental health has increased since our original publication in 2018, but in a way that is worryingly shallow. There is cause for celebration in seeing more writers like David Harewood[1] and Nadiya Hussein[2] speaking up in the public sphere about how racism has impacted their mental health. While social media is an important vessel for making these conversations public and accessible, platitudes such as #bekind do little in terms of structural impacts.

Despite the government's commissioned report from 2021 on Race and Ethnic Disparities denying the existence of systemic or institutional racism in the UK,[3] ethnic inequalities across society persist, and mental health is no exception.

At present, Black people are over four times more likely to be detained under the Mental Health Act than white people, and eight times more likely to be subject to a Community Treatment Order (CTO) – a legal order which allows you to be treated outside of hospital, in the community, but under strict conditions, like continuing treatment and living in a certain area.[4] Following an independent review of the Act in 2018, the government has proposed changes which would promote choice and reduce compulsion, but, notably, CTOs will still exist.[5]

We have also seen the expansion of the Serenity Integrated Mentoring (SIM) scheme, which brings in the police to reduce the demand on community mental health services by 'high intensity users'.[6] So, vulnerable people in distress are met by law enforcement rather than mental health professionals. The StopSIM Coalition, as well as professional bodies like the Royal College of Nurses, the Royal College of Psychiatrists, and the National Survivor User Network, have raised concerns about lack of consent, the sharing of clinical information with the police, and the criminalisation of distress, which many fear will only worsen racial inequalities.[7] While NHS England has agreed to review the scheme,[8] it is clear that the work to protect people of colour within the mental health services is far from over.

Doing the work

We have committed to being part of that reform work. It has been our privilege to witness the life the publication has had beyond its written form. Since the first edition, we have consistently been featured in outreach work across the UK, including multiple invited talks and workshops from academic conferences to grassroots organisations, and seen the book be added to NHS libraries, university syllabi, and placed on NHS mental health wards.

Following the anthology publication, we have been closely involved with multiple organisations devoted to improving mental health research and access to mental health support, particularly those that prioritise lived experience as a research method and in outcomes. This includes close work with organisations including the Wellcome Collection; the McPin Foundation; the Healthy Brains Global Initiative; the British Association for Behavioural and Cognitive Psychotherapies BAME counsellors working group; Southwark Council's Child and Adolescent Mental Health Services; and as two of the thirteen collaborators on the Cactus Foundation Researcher Mental Health survey report,[9] the largest global survey on researcher mental health and wellbeing with more than 13,000 participants globally.

We are also working with the Institute of Mental Health on their NEON (Narrative Experiences Online) study.[10] The study looks at how personal recovery stories may help those with psychosis and improve the way mental health workers support them. In particular, we are supporting their aim to 'focus on stories from people whose voices are seldom heard by mainstream cultures, and gathering them together to form the largest and most diverse online repository of mental health recovery stories in the world.'[11] We are delighted that some of the stories and experiences featured in *The Colour of Madness* have been an integral part of the study.

Structuring *The Colour of Madness*

In terms of the contents of this edition, the overall structure remains the same as in the first edition. Each colour chapter represents a different facet of mental health, guiding you through a kaleidoscopic collection of narratives, from passionate, rage-filled and resilient red; to orange, with racing, overwhelming thoughts to represent anxiety and mania; yellow to hold all the complexities and contradictions of hope. Green holds those pieces that focus on familial, and particularly filial, relationships; blue for our engagements with institutions, from clinical relationships in mental health institutions, to wider institutions such as the Home Office, immigration and refugee narratives, and academia. Indigo remains about depression and melancholy; violet is about experiences that are outside what we would traditionally think of as reality, and the polychrome chapter at the centre of the book draws this collection of narratives together with our contributors' artworks.

We encourage you to walk through *The Colour of Madness* at your own pace, taking the time to engage with each piece in whichever order you choose, remembering there is a whole person, an individual, behind each one. There is no single story of mental health, and here we present a kaleidoscope of experiences, for there are some who see the world in red, some who see the world in violet, and others who see the world somewhere in between these two ends of the spectrum.

Since its first publication, *The Colour of Madness* did exactly what we dreamed it would, reached the people it was meant to, and bolstered the work we anticipated it would. We hope that with the new life being given to it now, it will continue to touch people, and be part of the building of a more just world.

I return to my closing words from the original anthology, which remain as true now as the first time round: 'for all of us represented in this book, this cannot be a conclusion. It is closer to a beginning.'

Red

Sometimes, we see in red. We see through rage, we see through defiance.

He Was Red That Day

Andrés N. Ordorica

This is a story about Ismael and his great big adventure. Currently, he is sitting on an empty bench while the world gets on with its day. For whatever reason, he cannot. He has been this way for two months now.

No, he isn't dying, and no, he doesn't have cancer or anything like that. Quite frankly, Ismael is depressed, and he is not handling it well.

Self-imposed isolation has been his modus operandi these past few weeks, but Ismael realises how this could be exacerbating his sadness. He needs human contact, but in a controlled environment, among people who do not know him, or won't ask too many questions. Hence the whole sitting alone on a bench along the crowded River Thames. Near people, but invisible.

This plan was formulated by a mix of Reddit threads, his therapist's advice, and a few bottles of red wine. At some point last night, he reached a moment of clarity, turned to himself in the mirror and said, 'Fuck this recluse bullshit, Ismael. You need to get out of the flat tomorrow or else.' He wasn't prepared for the 'or else' and so here he is, outside his flat.

The truth is this unravelling has been a long time coming. In London, Ismael has rarely felt at ease. Cramped buses make his neck go red and hot. His collar will tighten around his throat whenever he rides the Underground – almost as if to kill him. The large crowds on the street give him headaches. The noise of the traffic makes sleep impossible. Everywhere pains him. This is not what he signed up for when he moved here a year ago for his postgrad degree.

He was used to a far simpler life, having grown up on his family's ranch in south Texas. But now, he is an urban cowboy battling the wild, wild metropolis. In a city where he assumed happiness would grow in abundance, but really is a pot of gold at the end of a rainbow he'll never find. So, Ismael has decided to spend the day alone, away from flatmates, co-workers, fellow students.

Ismael skipped work, took the Piccadilly line to Leicester Square and walked down to the river. He crossed over the Golden Jubilee bridge and clambered down the stairs towards the National Theatre. He looked upon the riverfront, long and wide, full of tourists and locals, and the thought of crowds overwhelmed him with exhaustion.

So, he is seeking refuge on his favourite bench. The bench he comes to whenever he is stressed, sad or angry, which seems to be more and more lately. One day, it will be dedicated posthumously to him with a little brass sign:

> THIS BENCH SERVES AS A MEMORY OF THE SANITY
> THAT WAS LOST BY ISMAEL ESCOBEDO –
> A MILLENNIAL WHO COULD NO LONGER COPE WITH
> THIS GARBAGE-HEAP OF A PLANET.

Sometimes, Ismael's anxiety comes on like some wave ready to wash over him and pin him to the ocean floor. Letting him slowly drown in painful death. Sometimes, he can see the anxiety edging closer to him, and sometimes, it just appears out of nowhere, ready to ruin everything like an uninvited party guest.

He closes his eyes and wonders whether he is just another 'snowflake' having a mental breakdown or if something deeper is at play. Something that he should really be worried about. The city is doing this, he tells himself. *It's you, London, not me.*

As the clouds move out of the way and the sun heats up his skin, Ismael is reminded how not all is terrible. Sometimes, urban life can be beautiful, and London a place worth living in. Even the dirty Thames has its moments.

Water has always transfixed Ismael. He spent his childhood in the water, constantly diving and splashing about. Whether in the pond on his family ranch, the municipal pool, or summer holidays by the Gulf of Mexico. The brown and green water of his youth was both disgusting and alluring, like the Thames. But no matter the colour of the water, there was sunshine and freedom, at least in those memories. That is what he needs, *freedom*, an escape of some sort. But to where?

'Ahem.'

God, is that you?

'Ahhheeeemmm.'

No, not God. But it is someone. Someone who is clearing their throat. Someone who is trying to tell him something. Ismael opens his eyes to see who it is – an older woman, fifty plus, weighed down by numerous bags. There are literally two open benches in his direct line of vision, but she continues to shuffle closer.

'This here is my seat. Move!' she instructs him – a slight accent to her accent mapping out a history far larger than this city, this country even.

He is taken aback by her abrupt and curt tone. He has always thought of old women as warm and kind. But she is brash and forthright.

'Ahem, I said; move.'

He sits up and moves over. The old lady whacks him with

her shopping trolley by accident, or she plays it off that way. She sits down and starts digging through one of her many bags. His peaceful aura is gone, and so is his solitude. She retrieves a can of Jamaican ginger beer, opens it, and takes a big gulp, and some of it trickles down her chin. She lets out a burp and then begins searching her things once more. She finds an emery board and files down one of her nails. They are long and shellacked, decorated with rhinestones and painted with what he gathers to be a tropical design. She lets out another loud burp. He cannot help but laugh, but she pays him no mind.

'Can I ask you a question?' he is surprised by himself. He hates talking to strangers, but he knows he must speak to her.

'What the hell are you bugging me for?'

'Ugh, rude!'

She just stares at him, dumbfounded that he is still trying to talk to her. Her face is uninviting, but he persists.

'How do you get the world to just do what you want?'

'What?'

'There are literally two free benches next to us, yet you got even me to move.'

She rolls her eyes, desperate for Ismael to shut the hell up.

'Hello? I asked you a question – and politely, I might add.'

'Man, you're annoying as fuck.'

'Probably,' he concedes.

'My method, if you must know . . . is I simply don't give two shits what anyone thinks of me. Understand?'

People pass them by in twos and threes, deep in their own conversations.

'This is my bench, by the way. That's why you moved.'

In this moment, those passing by know nothing of their struggle to claim ownership of this city property.

'It's mine. But, whatever,' Ismael offers.

She tuts, a slight smirk appearing on her face. She then starts filing her nails again. A good minute or so passes before she stops and looks up at Ismael, deep into his eyes.

'You can't let anyone drag you down, do you get me?'

Is it possible she is reading his mind?

'You're too cute, baby boy, to look that sad and pathetic.'

She holds her stare, and he can't help but be drawn to her honey-gold eyes.

'Thank you . . .'

'Candace.'

'Ismael.'

'You're welcome, Ismael. Now, please shut up and let me have some bloody peace and quiet!'

Ismael does just that. He gathers his things and scurries away. Cantankerous Candace is now responsible for keeping watch of their bench and Ismael, well, he is tasked with continuing today's journey.

He should be at work but is taking a 'mental health day'. At least that's how he'll explain it when he turns his phone back on. How many messages will there be? How many missed calls and urgent emails exist in the ether right now, waiting for him to press the power button? He has all the power and not an ounce of desire to find out. So, he heads for the Tate Modern. Home to such pretty and strange-looking works of art.

He enters via the long ramp and chooses to run down it. A group of six-year-old school children follow his lead, breaking into a stampede and screaming at the tops of their lungs. Their teachers and chaperones desperately struggle to wrangle up the class. He high-fives a few of them before walking away. A cloud of happiness and serotonin hangs above the mayhem. He then takes the lift to the top of the museum, where there is a cafe overlooking the riverbank. He decides to treat himself to a glass of wine. The art can wait.

'A Merlot, please,' he says to the cute cafe worker.

He is handed a plastic cup and bottle, which he pours out before recycling. He takes a giant gulp of wine, and it burns his throat. Slow down, Ismael, he warns himself.

He notices a free table outside and beats two yummy mummies to it. The mums give him evil eyes as they stroll off in defeat. He lights a cigarette and takes in the view. The dome of St Paul's looks beautiful even with all those ugly buildings crowding it. Its holiness is evident in its careful design.

He remembers going there for evensong after his grandmother passed away a few months ago. He'd lit a candle and mumbled some words and a prayer from childhood. She'd have appreciated the candle and the 'Hail Mary'. He'd closed his eyes, taken in the choir music, and silently cried that day. Ismael opens his eyes to his present, but a pain still lingers inside no matter how much time has passed.

'It's getting a bit cold, no?' he observes to no one in particular.

He downs his wine and begins his search for the painting at the centre of today's adventure. One by Rothko, part of his 'Red' series for the Four Seasons. It was a painting that had moved him as a child. He needs to be moved once more. To prove to himself that he can feel more than just anger and sadness. When he was a child, Ismael wanted to paint his room red, but his parents chose blue, and blue he became. Nevertheless, a red ember burnt inside him like a pilot light waiting to explode.

Ismael mindlessly walks down the stairs to the fifth floor before remembering that his painting is somewhere on the second floor. He heads to the escalators, going down three storeys, not aiding his search with a map but his deep intuition. This painting is his kindred spirit calling him home. *He will find it.*

The Tate is much busier than he anticipated for a weekday. Far busier than he remembers when entering, before drinking his red wine, before being so lost.

'Live and learn,' he mutters to himself.

He could make this all easier by just asking a gallery attendant for directions. But he no longer has the energy to interact with other people. There's a free bench, his second of the day, so he decides to rest for a moment and gather his thoughts.

Galleries and museums allow for a certain level of anonymity. People don't come to talk, people don't come to be seen; they come for the art. The mesmerising, confusing, and sometimes pretentious, art. There is a code of ethics one undertakes when visiting a gallery. He enjoys the safety of being near people but free of the weight of conversation.

He closes his eyes to concentrate on his breathing. Just his breathing. He scans his body to get a sense of his nostrils, lungs, feet pressing on the ground. His therapist told him that mindfulness works that way. Like a dialogue with the body.

'Excuse me,' says a squeaky little voice.

A small hand nudges his kneecap, forcing his eyes open. There is a cute little girl, no more than eight, standing in front of him.

He takes a deep breath, readying himself for whatever drama he is about to get into, 'Yes? Can I help you?'

'Umm . . . I'm lost.'

'Sorry. Did you say you're "lost"?'

She pauses nervously, 'Yes. I need help.'

Her lips start quivering, and he notices how puffy her face looks. Snot runs down her nose. He realises that she has been crying. He looks around for other adults, but no one pays either of them any attention.

'Are you here with your mom or dad?'

'No.'

'Who are you with?'

'My grandpa. But I don't know where he is. He went to the toilet, but I can't find him.'

'Okay, okay. It will be fine,' he says, hoping to reassure them both.

She wipes her nose with the sleeve of her coat.

'Thank you.'

'My name is Ismael.'

'Feather. My name is Feather,' she says, extending her hand like a little grown-up.

'It's nice to meet you, Feather. Okay, let's see if we can go find a nice gallery worker to help us find your grandad.'

They head to an exhibition entry to speak to one of the attendants; a young-looking art student, probably hoping to run the gallery one day.

'Tickets, please!'

'Oh, no. We aren't here to see the exhibition.'

'Okay, well this queue is for ticket holders or those who wish to purchase tickets, only.'

Ismael tries to not wear his annoyance so obviously on his face.

'Well, yes, but you see, my little friend here is l-o-s-t.'

'Lost! But isn't she with you?'

Ismael takes in a deep breath and counts to five.

'Well, actually my friend, Feather, is visiting the gallery with her grandfather, and they seem to have broken away from each other by accident.'

'I see now. Well, not to worry, we can definitely help you, Feather.'

'Thank you, miss.'

'You're welcome. Now, what's your grandad's name?'

'Kwesi Richardson.'

'Very good. Now, where was the last place you saw Mr Rich-ardson? I mean, your grandad?'

'He went to the toilet and asked me to wait for him outside in the hallway.'

'Can you remember what floor that was on?'

'The top floor,' she says, smiling like she has won a quiz.

'Great, Feather, that's really helpful. I just need to make a few calls to some of my colleagues now. I won't be more than a few minutes.'

Ismael wonders how often the staff get trained on helping lost people – lost children – find their family members. Might she be able to help his lost soul, too?

'I hope that he isn't angry,' Feather says out of nowhere, guilt in her voice.

'Your grandad? No, he is probably just a bit worried.'

'I shouldn't have wandered off.'

'No, but it happens sometimes.'

'Still, I shouldn't have,' she says, looking up. He smiles faintly and pats her on the head.

Ismael has never been good with kids. At least, he has never had ample opportunity to improve upon his skills. None of his siblings or friends have kids. His interaction with children has been minimal up until this point. Paternal warmth does not come easy to him.

'Everything will be fine,' he says, unsure who needs to hear it.

He watches as the attendant speaks quickly into her walkie, looking over at them every few words. Her face is painted with worry, and he knows something is up. *Dear God, please don't let anything be wrong.*

She walks towards them at a brisk pace.

'Feather, do you mind helping me out for a minute?' asks the attendant.

'No, I don't mind.'

'Do you think you can sit at this desk here with my friend Betty? She could use your help checking the tickets while I speak to your new friend.'

'Okay, that sounds fun,' she looks up to Ismael for his approval. He nods.

'Betty, this is Feather. Feather, Betty.'

'Nice to meet you, Feather,' says a woman nearer to Ismael's age. Her accent broad and Scottish.

'Nice to meet you, Miss.'

'Betty, me and this gentleman will only be a minute.'

She forcefully grabs Ismael by the hand and drags him about ten feet away from the exhibition entry. He knows something must be wrong by how erratically she is behaving. She takes in a deep breath. This can't be good.

'It seems Mr Richardson has had a heart attack.'

'Holy shit. What do you mean?' he asks in a low but urgent voice.

'That's why Feather couldn't find him. That's why he never came out of the toilet. She must have been waiting for a long time.'

'I'm so confused.'

'Well, apparently one of my colleagues called emergency services over two hours ago to help a man that had taken ill in the disabled toilet on the sixth floor.'

'Oh, my God, and you're certain it's him?'

'Yes, we're confident. Feather's mother is on her way now.'

'This poor girl,' he says while watching her from afar.

'Feather's parents were notified that Mr Richardson was taken to St Thomas', and it was only when they showed up that they realised their daughter was missing. My colleagues were trying to locate her around the same time she found you.'

'Is he going to be okay?'

'I don't have any information. Just that her mother is on her way.'

He stops paying attention to her and looks over at Feather, who seems to be having the time of her life working the ticket counter. Feather and Betty are like two peas in a pod. Betty handles the ticket purchases, and Feather scans the visitors in. The scanning device looks comically huge in her childish hands.

'What are we going to tell Feather?'

'Simply that her mum is on the way to get her and that her grandad was feeling a bit unwell, but that her parents will take her to see him as soon as they can.'

'Okay; I don't know if I will be of any more use.'

'You don't have to stay if you don't want to.'

'I just don't want to complicate the situation.'

'You've been great. Honestly, God knows what could have happened had you not found her.'

'Thanks. I mean, it was her. She found me. I didn't do anything special.'

He doesn't want to agitate Feather by saying goodbye, and so he just disappears into the crowd. He feels a bit strange, but still needs to see that Rothko painting. He continues deep into the galleries of the second floor. It is nearby; he can feel it.

It was during his sixth-grade art class when he first saw it. He would have been a few years older than Feather. Probably around eleven. He remembers how awesome it looked on the projector screen. It was as if some giant red wave was going to wash over his class at any moment. He got close, dangerously close to the screen. His teacher thought Ismael was just being disruptive, but he wasn't, honestly. He just wanted to see as much red as possible. He still needs to.

* * *

Each room is full of other artists: Hockney, Rauschenberg. He can tell his Manet from his Monet, but his Rothko eludes him. He passes the melting clocks of Dalí and Tracey Emin's self-portraits, but none of them contain the red he needs. There are sculptures and installations, which are impressive, but irrelevant. They are not the things that could bring him the joy he longs for.

Where is it? Has it left him? Like his grandmother, like past boyfriends, like how he left his life in the United States? Boarded a plane, changed address, and started over.

'Please, please, come back!' he begs it.

Does anyone understand how much he needs this red?

He walks a bit more, but it is starting to all feel pointless. He can't fix everything with silence and distance. He can't put a Band-Aid over his heart and expect all to be fine. He lets his mind switch on to autopilot, lets his leg muscles direct his feet, and pushes on despite the sense of purposelessness hanging above him.

The crowds move like a wave, pulling in and out. Children giggle in groups while older kids take pictures on their phones for Instagram, TikTok, Twitter. All these selfies being uploaded for likes and shares and comments. They're like a school of fish swimming from one side of the room to the other, depending on who has the funniest photos. But eventually, they part like the Red Sea as their teacher ushers them along. Finally, some room to breathe.

The gallery is too huge, too overwhelming, too bloody full of art. Maybe the painting really has moved. A piece of art as transient as Ismael, always moving, always occupying new and unfamiliar spaces. On loan, gifted, purchased . . . always by the generous donation, endowment, inheritance, betrothal of some dead aristocrat. But, what about the common man who cannot gift anything? What can he leave behind? These thoughts soon sadden him further.

Ismael is just going through the motions at this point. The day has been long, a waste even. He won't find it. Instead, he turns his phone back on. He should have been at work three hours ago. Fifteen missed calls, twenty emails, eleven text messages.

Where are you? Getting kind of late! The boss is freaking out and I don't know what to say? Are you dead?

Hope you're excited for your birthday dinner! Hey, we still on for tonight?

¡Feliz cumpleaños, mijo! Dad and I hope you can FaceTime soon.

Hey, I thought we were meeting a half-hour ago? Where you at . . . did I do something wrong?

No, it was him. It was Ismael that did the wrong thing. He is sorry for being a bad friend, selfish son, distant colleague, and neglectful lover. He puts the phone back in his pocket. He wants to leave. He needs to find the exit. He wants to disappear. The exit sign finally is there in front of him. Illuminating. Green. Just a sign. Not an art piece. Nothing ironic here. Just a sign to tell him where to go, what to do, how to escape.

'You need to calm down, Ismael.'

His head starts to spin, or is it the room? He struggles toward another bench and sits himself down, his third one today.

'Close your eyes, breathe; don't have a panic attack.'

1, 2, 3, 4, 5, 6, 7, 8, 9, 10.

'Take in a deep breath. Exhale using your mouth.'

1, 2, 3, 4, 5, 6, 7, 8, 9, 10.

He repeats until he is ready to open his eyes and . . . *there it is* . . . now breathe in . . . *but it's standing right in front of him.* And breathe out . . . *well, not standing but hanging* . . . and breathe in once more . . . *that's what paintings do.*

'Hello, old friend. It's me. I've missed you.'

Ismael stands up and inches closer to the painting – dangerously close. He lets the red wash over him like he always wanted. How beautiful it looks in the dimly lit room free from others. How cleansing the burgundies are for his soul, like warm blood pumping through his body, keeping him alive – 'sanguine', he will name it, that elusive shade.

As he takes it in, Ismael remembers what it is to not be sad all the time. There is much more to life than sadness; there is joy and love, which he deserves, and can give to others. This painting is a reminder of how much he appreciates his life: the green of the sea, the blue of the sky, the yellow of a daisy's centre. But right now, he *sees* red and *is* red. To Ismael, red is happiness, and happiness is exactly what it's like to be standing in a quiet gallery in a city of millions of people just trying to get on with their day.

Resolute

Nisha Damji

I'm not resilient, I'm told.
Because it hurts me when they tear me down
With their eyes, words
And bitter judgement.
I am at fault, I'm told,
because I am not like them.
My hurt and my pain is pathologised
because I am other,
because I am a stranger,
because I am Brown,
And I won't bend.

Needle Reclamations

Tajah Hamilton

When I looked at my body, all I saw were the multitude of phantom hands laid on me.

With every prick of the tattoo needle, I crafted my rebirth, dextrous hands smoothing and raising my clay form.

Every tattoo was a reclamation.

Every glance in the mirror from that first smooth line onwards was silent protest.

A protest against a body that, still, at times feels those phantom hands and shudders, disgust fused into my veins.

A body that was claimed as belonging to another when we can't fucking claim people, and it KNEW that, the mind connected to it knew that, and yet it was placed under house arrest for three years.

House arrest with a one-way mirror, witnessing the abduction of my Black body that was subjected to multitudes of terror, during – and after I left.

My mind still feels like it's undergoing a heart massage.

These are the scars ink has made occult.

But now, all I see are images of strength.

Four hours of needlework for four years of my life spent
spiralling – dandelion seed again in flight.

Twenty-five minutes for the month where suicide plagued todos
de mi pensamientos.

One hour for the year I found my direction, and colour entered
my life again – where I allowed myself to pursue my interests
and give my love to the people who were beyond deserving, and
to feel it myself, because I deserved it too.

My tattoos remind me that it's not just leaving that's strong, it's
dealing with the aftermath of 'what could've been' if you'd left
sooner.

My tattoos remind me that all of my moments from now on will
be concrete decisions forged on the back of self-belief.

My revolutions against my mind's sometimes-ish preoccupation
with sending me down a rabbit hole that I can only escape from
by eating myself.

The eternal reminder that I'm now free from my cell and
planting roots like I hoped I would when I first planted my tree
on my chest.

No, next time

Jess Brough

On the night I was celebrated
in a room of strangers,
someone close obscured my name
and chose violence, when there was longing
waiting in consenting hands.

That's not to say it's too late
to taste the shape of an invitation, rescinded.
Give me a prize so I can speak it next time,

And you may never hear a sigh of relenting.
That's not to say the cool wind against my skin
does not make me think of love in autumn,
nor does two shadows in a doorway indifferent to spies.

And still, my body trembles
with the nearness of another.
But that's not to say I feel safe in October.

Safety exists on the wings of a promise
and splinters under pressure,
brought down to its knees.

That's not to say my hands won't find
a path that leads to heaven.
And the thrill that seeks her knowing touch,
won't find thunder
in caring palms.

Orange

And sometimes, we see in orange. In desperate
thoughts and conflicting wants, in panic and
anxiety.

Boiling Kettles

Louisa Adjoa Parker

An endless loop of panic:
will the house burn down
while I'm away? Will it still
be standing when I return?
Will I return? Are the hair straighteners
unplugged, the cooker turned off?
Will water pipes freeze and burst?
Will burglars get in?
I think of ghosts of irons
flat-down on burning boards,
of kettles boiling, on repeat.

Your Problem is You Worry Too Much

Ruvimbo Gumbochuma

head.
Why do you pray every night if you know God is not real? You
say 'God forbid' while knocking on wood. Your words echo what
your mother said, and her mother, and her mother before.

mouth.
Why does tomorrow haunt you and sit on your throat every
time you speak? Why do you grind your teeth and gums until
they bleed?

chest.
Why can't you sleep when it's as easy as a deep breath? Or a
kiss from your girlfriend? Or a hug from your sister?

hands.
Why are you scared all the time? You crack your knuckles then
crack them more. You remember someone told you it causes
arthritis.

legs.

Why are you angry when your brother forgets to call back? You remember when he stole sweets from Dad's shop and ran until he fell and bruised his knees.

Why do you plan a funeral whenever you're sick?

Why are you scared?

The Mice in the Walls

Dania Quadri

I can hear a desperate
scurrying in the walls,
strange sounds grate against
my eardrum: a serrated knife
sawing into cardboard at a
million angles, sawdust
streams form under me.

I rouse, kick off the quilt,
stand tall on my bed, rap
on the wall. The scurrying
quietens, momentarily halts.
But as soon as I lay my head
back down on the pillow,
eyes gazing into an imaginary sky;

the mice are crawling
between the walls again.
I try to block out the sounds,
but I'm alone; they envelop me.
I wonder if our fears –

founded / unfounded, lurk
between the walls as well;

quickly quieten at a rap,
but soon entrench the folds
of our minds and grow louder
and louder still. I turn on
the lamp to deceive them,
clinging onto the warmth
of my little light, praying

it will keep the mice away.
But where would they go?
Maybe the creatures of habit,
scurry along the same route
between the cardboard walls
in this cardboard house
because they'd rather be safe

than brave the unscripted.
Maybe they see no obvious
way of leaving, so they infest
the walls, make it their home.
If only, the rap persisted
/ light burnt down the walls,
they would finally scurry away.

Lost

Corinne Crosbourne
aka 'thewomanistwords'

I have lost my mother tongue;
fragmented, broken, splintered words remain.
I have lost clear brown eyes,
fogged by History's shame.
I have lost my direction,
the stars no longer shine.
I have lost a family tree,
its branches dead, entwined.

I have lost a nation,
and how to say my name.
I have lost a history,
my people brutalised and claimed.

But I have gained a wisdom,
sure and deep and true.
I've learned to bite the hand that fed me,
and turn my back on you.

Pomegranate

Zeena Yasin

your brain is like a pomegranate
some of the seeds are ripe and fresh
many others crushed
their contents trickling to the other parts of your mind
they stick and stick
stick and stick
you try to clean out your mind
removing a lot of its contents
until your brain is all
fresh and clean.
But now you have to start anew
having forgotten an entire lifetime

Ramblings of the Scarred

Danielle DZA Osajivbe-Williams

*I am a two-sided coin, which possesses both visibility and
    invisibility.*
*In this land, as other, I adjust to standards I wasn't made
    to meet.*
Intergenerational trauma is embedded in my DNA.
Blackmail, black cat, black sheep; repeat.

I didn't understand the relationship between Blackness and my
identity until the age of seven. After returning from a three-
year stint living in my grandmother's birthplace Barbados, I
was suddenly submerged back into the Black-British experience.
This meant questioning whether my newly observed rejection at
the hands of white people was because I didn't look like them. I
remember observing a Catholic priest reluctantly place communion bread on my father's lips.

Skip to age eleven. I am in a majority-Black school, only it's
not like Barbados. I don't feel I belong. I am the tallest in my year,
the lowest year of the school. My self-worth is refracted through
the perceptions of others: their perceptions are not great. Africa
is a dirty word even to me, yet I am half-Nigerian. I have internalised the view of Africa as a country rather than a continent. A
country with famine, ugliness, and corruption.

The self-hatred I have internalised worsens once I realise I am viewed as African by others. My cheekbones high, skin dark – I have no proof of West Indian heritage. I feel isolated from the Black British community.

Skip forward to age fourteen. I am an overweight, depressed, anxious, angst-ridden teen. I isolate myself from the Black-British community. I despise all of my family and listen to alternative music. My racial identity feels unfamiliar. I am now an emo kid; a non-conforming, vegetarian, coconut, goth. All the anxiety and paranoia I have felt before this age is irrelevant, because now, not only am I on edge all the time, I am filled with a silent rage which seeks to tear me apart from the inside.

I no longer view beauty as belonging to West Indians. Instead, beauty is coloured contacts, coloured hair extensions, skinny frames, and alternative fashion. I still want to be me, dark skin and all, but with white beauty standards. All the images I look at are of girls who don't look like me.

Throughout all of this I am cutting myself to cope. I lash out at my single mum behind closed doors while simultaneously presenting as bubbly and happy to the outside world. When I finally try to get help through the NHS, my mum is horrified. As a mental health support worker, she sees first-hand the dispro-portionate number of Black males in her facility requiring legal drugs to manage their diagnoses, their eyes pleading with her to save them – her kin. Confused and overwhelmed, I fail to respond to the NHS letter.

I remember being sixteen and not knowing my true emotions as a result of faking all the time. Sometimes, I felt tearful when I wanted to laugh: I had tried to be strong for so long that my body had had enough.

I remember thinking self-harm was not something Black girls did. I felt more isolated from my community: a coconut who dealt with things like a white girl. I desperately wanted to belong some-where. I was unable to be honest with others about my difficulties. I didn't feel that I was important enough, and my friendships were too precious for me to risk behaving like myself.

I don't know how to be honest with doctors either. I don't fully understand myself, and I don't trust them. I can share the tip of the iceberg, the front-page symptoms on Google. Not my lack of hygiene, my worries about being poor, my discreet suicide attempts made to look accidental, or my laxative reliance.

I miss A-level exams because I think I am a failure. I can't cross the road properly from overthinking. I am always away with the fairies. I avoid places where I have been spooked by someone or something. I constantly dwell on past conversations.

Skip forward to eighteen. I am at a new college studying psychology. I have lost weight and feel more confident, convinced that this is the cure. But I am still anxious. I self-medicate with weed. I am doing well at college, so it truly must be the healing of the nations.

I still struggle in social situations, feeling crippling pain and paranoia when going to meet people, but a fear of missing out when I don't. I am going back to the doctors, giving them self-diagnoses of personality disorders. I am viewed as a hypo-chondriacal student. I know what is wrong with me; help me.

Skip forward to nineteen. I have made it to university. The panic attack, which impacted one of my exam grades, couldn't stop me. I am with the boy I've spent years pining over. I am coming out of my shell. My mental health is still deteriorating, and I receive counselling through university and then the NHS. Scared about the deterioration of my health, I plead for early-intervention help. I want counselling. This fails. I am put on antidepressants. The cycle of weed, and then alcohol, self-harm and emotional eating continues.

Things improve when I find out about community counselling initiatives. I always knew I just needed a counsellor, one that was not limited to six sessions, where I would feel safe to go deeper than surface-level. In this space I am able to confront the intersection of my identity; race, gender, class, and my mental health.

I learned to lift my voice, to speak up about these issues and not suffer in silence. It was both empowering and reassuring to meet like-minded people, some of which are from the BAME community who are able to share their experiences too. Volunteering as a mental health advocate was a useful way for me to do this, but also opening up to friends and family has been liberating.

I have learned that there is a long-standing tradition for Black communities to feel the need to be strong: everything must look pristine to outsiders. I spent a lot of time feeling isolated from the Black community, and as a result, I failed to see that my mental health issues were inextricably linked to my racial identity.

For all the black sheep, who can't always see their Black is magic: I share this in the hope that you may feel less alone. It takes strength to let your guard down. To love and care for yourself in a space which sees you as polar. We are built to survive, but we must strive to thrive.

Postscript

When I first wrote this piece and agreed to participate in this anthology, I am not sure I fully understood the ramifications of revealing a raw and, for the most part, unfiltered account of my experiences with mental health. I was just beginning my training as a counsellor and psychotherapist, where we learn to be authentic without being too transparent about who we are. 'It is not about us', we are told. And so, I was terrified about what it would mean to me, my training and practice to reveal this unfettered and accessible knowledge about my challenges, my perspectives on life from a retrospective view, without apology.

At the same time, sharing my experiences felt necessary. It was necessary for the younger me, whose story I was telling, and those like her who had yet to find the words. As healing practitioners in mental health industries, we often reinforce unhealthy and unrealistic projections. We reinforce power dynamics where we are peddled as 'expert' without being able to relay our own human experience – one we are still on a journey towards grappling with.

Revisiting this piece for this revised edition was difficult. I believe that part of this is because I now view and understand these experiences in different ways - there are new words I would use to talk about what was happening. Terms like internalised racism, race-based trauma, internalised fatphobia, disordered eating – I was aware of many of these concepts before, but fully accepting them as features of my own history has been harder to fathom. I would like to share some of my learning, as I have come to understand these experiences, the impact on my body as a consequence not fitting the status quo, adjusting to 'a standard I wasn't *made to meet*'.

Working somatically (relating to bodily experience) and learning about trauma-informed therapies which take account of non-verbal responses to stress and trauma has been profoundly necessary for supporting my health. Where possible, take note of your gait and the sensational and emotional qualities of your experience whenever you are in different environments. Take note of tension or tightness, soreness, temperature, ease, softness, alertness. Notice the places you feel like you can be you; this could be when you're alone, with trusted, supportive friends, or with a therapist/healer. Now compare this with spaces you feel the need to perform in, hide, contort, code-switch, the spaces where you may feel more aware of yourself as 'different' to others. This is an invitation to shift, unfurl, breathe, and regulate if it feels safe to do so in the moment. If it doesn't, schedule in time for where you can do so in safety. When we don't notice, often we don't shift, and we become perpetually stuck in the contorted space. If you are yet to find the spaces where you can be you, yet to know what 'being you' feels like, or unable to notice the sensations and emotional qualities, I want to say that this is an invitation you can keep revisiting with patience and care. I want to say well done for doing your best. There is so much that our bodies do on autopilot with the view to keeping us alive. It is very rare we are invited to take notice.

Finally, ancestral wisdom has been a guiding light for me on the journey of wellness. Since qualifying as a therapist, my journey has taken me on a search for ancestral and spiritual healing practices. I have a drive to bring Black narratives, African narratives of healing to the forefront, assisting in the dissemination of healing technologies of past/present/future. I believe that as well as intergenerational trauma, we have intergenerational medicine embedded in our DNA. There are those who came before us and thrived. We have been here for a very long time, long before the narratives we are told is our history, Black history. A history outside of survival, struggle, and resistance. Tap in. This can be through communing with elders and asking them what has kept them well, researching the healing traditions of ancestral lands, building an ancestral altar to connect with and elevate those ancestors, known and unknown, who displayed the traits you would like to embody, such as resilience and joy.

To end, I wish to say that I hope that this anthology and the intentions of my sharing have had the desired outcome. I hope it has given a voice to some of the experiences those of our community have felt. I hope that it has paved the way for health industries and institutions to listen to us and challenge their own biases. Whether struggling or not, I wish peace, protection, and proper care to all of us in communities marginalised by western societies due to race and/or ethnicities – especially those with further marginalised experiences due to disability, weight distribution, gender, sexuality, and shade. Finally, I offer gratitude and appreciation to Dr Samara Linton, Rianna Walcott and all the contributors to this body of work for doing what needs to be done.

Yellow

At other times, we see in yellow, where the sun both
warms and burns; the complexity of hope.

Little Birds Hope

Caroline

Two birds, both one and the same.
One flies high over treetops, wings spread, caressing the
  clouds.
The other, caged with clipped wings, sings, weeping tears
  of joy at the promise of its future.

Sunshine Girl

Ailsa Fineron

Feeling hurt. Wanting to scream, but the fear of being heard clogs my throat, plugging it with petrol-soaked rags, gagging on words crawling up and down my oesophagus. Fingers form a fist clenching around my lungs, squeezes the tongues I have grown, and the grip tastes of burnt coffee. The promise of something delicious coating your teeth with bitterness, so that when you smile, you smile through disappointment. Everyone can see, but only if they look. I understand.

I am the sunshine girl. An easy stream to cool your feet in, something pleasant to dip into. You do not want to see the depths where I have drowned many times; nor do I. Still, I go diving, looking for pearls, for gems grown from choking dust. Once you've been pulled down here you cannot come up for air. So let go. Let the weight of your heart turned to iron pull you down. Don't fight it. Drowning is quicker if you attempt to inhale. Let the weight of your heart turned to an anchor drop through you.

Release your hands from each other. Broken fingers would leave you unable to write and then what would you do? Speaking is not an option for now. Use your words. Use the craft you practised in the hours when the cars sleep. Picking adjectives from the hand-carved, hand-smoothed treasure box under your bed, trying out each one until you hear the click of the right fit. Remember the satisfaction of capturing an elusive flying-cloud-mood and preserving its complexities on paper. Use your words.

Reach out and others reach back. Their messages make you laugh, cry, turn you to a marble statue, polished and shining. Warm hands on your shoulders, in your hair, framing your face, because they know why and how you are beautiful. And since you cannot see it for yourself you let them show you. This time is different. Reach out and others reach back. You are learning, and I am proud.

Now is the time for resting. For walking home. Unlacing boots with blood-filled fingers, sitting on the side of the bath and running swollen feet under cold water until you can dance again. Sitting in the cool of the living room, letting the bright lights fade to black on the back of my eyelids. Now is the time for gentleness. Yes, there is fear of loss, terror of another time spent in something deeper than sadness. But the best you can do is be gentle. Feed yourself. Lie in warm water hearing the rain fall on glass. Inhale and help yourself to float. You are in a still lake in the cotton-soft night, glowing blue sky, the breeze, and ripples on your skin the breath of a world that reminds you of your worth. Float half-submerged: body in transparent ink, lips just kissed by air, your arms have nothing to hold in this moment. Float for now in the comfort of knowing the depths below and above you.

Postscript

I wrote this five years ago, in 2016, aged twenty-two. Reading it back is like reading another person's words. As you can see, I was beginning to cultivate some self-compassion, and I'm pleased to say that now I have a huge amount of love for both my present self and this twenty-two-year-old me. It's taken a long time though, and has been the hardest work I've ever done: to go from believing I was wrong and not even being able to recognise shame to now responding to shame with self-compassion and allowing others to care for me too.

I have person-centred psychodynamic therapy and the trauma-informed approach to thank for this, along with the love and company of many beautiful people. I have been privileged enough to access long-term private therapy for the past four and a half years. My journey has led me from medicalising mental health issues to a much more holistic view that takes into account systemic issues, trauma (systemic and interpersonal) and the importance of relationships. In 2016, I found the label of bipolar II validating: it helped me believe I did deserve help, but it also meant I sometimes fell into the trap of trying to fulfil my diagnosis and being told that I would always be this way. I am pleased to say that 2016 was also the last time I had an episode. My work as a support worker in complex trauma, independent mental health advocate, and counsellor training has reinforced how important it is to view ourselves and others as complex, nuanced and ever-changing individuals, each with a unique history.

I dream of a world where everyone is able to ask for and access the help they need, as I have – be it emotional, financial, housing etc. – without having to prove their suffering through a label or reaching an externally determined 'crisis point'. We have a long way to go, but I am hopeful that things are changing. My generation may be sneered at as 'snowflakes', but I see us as a generation of people who are unwilling to put up with the trauma and pain of the world that has been handed to us. I believe that the work of healing ourselves and healing society are interlinked. It heartens me to see so many people now facing their pain, processing it and protesting it.

The Stigma of Suicide

Kalwinder Singh Dhindsa

In South Asian communities, the man is seen as the head of the household. So much is expected of him from the instant he takes on the responsibility to provide for his family. My father was a proud and gentle man who always tried to do his best for those closest to him. My father was a good man. He was not a criminal; he did not commit a crime. He did not commit suicide.

My father, Mohinder Singh Dhindsa, died by suicide on 1 March 2006. My father died from a mental illness that had corrupted his mind, silencing him forever. His death also silenced many more around him who were also deeply affected by his death.

For a long time after his death, I tried to avoid using the word 'suicide'. However, when it would slip into conversation, I would precede it with 'commit'. In time, I realised that 'commit' was not an appropriate word to use. Once upon a time, suicide was a crime in this nation before it was abrogated. I refuse to use this term anymore as it is unfair to the victims of suicide and their families and loved ones left behind for them to carry this extra burden of implied criminality.

Suicide stops people talking. Whether it is the person who has just taken their own life, or the loved ones bereaved and left behind to pick up the pieces. Lack of engagement with the bereaved is a serious problem in the Punjabi community, due to the apparent fear of upsetting close family, just not being able to broach the subject, or simply not knowing what to say. Another factor is the issue of shame and dishonour that is deeply instilled in the personas of Punjabi people and their culture. All these factors further diminish the good memories of the loved one who has passed on, and as they are no longer talked about they could be forgotten about forever.

Immediately after my father's death, I knew that I could never allow my memories of him to be lost in time. Therefore, I decided to write down all the feelings and memories I still had of him in my life, up to that point. They had to be written down for posterity; to be kept safe from the fear of one day losing them altogether, should my own mind also be corrupted in the same manner as my father's.

Suicide stops people in their tracks. On 1 March 2006 that was definitely the case for me. It took me a long while to finally get back on track; an uncertain journey that eventually saw me on the straight and narrow. It began almost nine years later when I heard about what led to the death of Robin Williams. The symptoms that he had been experiencing seemed to very much mirror those of my father's – the hallucinations in particular. The phantom aches and pains. As well as his confused state and issues with his memory. I now think of Robin Williams as the man who set me free, the man who provided me with a form of closure and an acceptance of what happened. This freedom gave me the strength to do my utmost to help others who have also travelled a similar path.

It was difficult to talk to anyone at the time; a cloak of silence seemed to have masked all attempts to understand why my father's death occurred. Religion mixed with custom, soaked in culture. Suicide was taboo, a stigma to be avoided at all costs. Eventually, I began to seek some professional help. Thankfully, I was referred to a mental health therapist who helped me set foot on the road to happiness. A person who listened without prejudice, unblemished by society's taboos. Pain was the motivator for my change; an opportunity to question my life and move on. There had been no time to stop and contemplate the darkness. I needed to be distracted. Thankfully, writing came to my rescue.

> During my darkest moments I still had dreams of completing my story and one day releasing it as a book. As much as my doubts plagued me, thinking that I might never finish it. I refused to give up and kept pushing myself onwards by telling myself that my story needed to be told and only I could complete it. Nobody else was going to write it for me. I owed that to my father to finish our shared story, to continue to keep his memory alive.
>
> (Extract from: *My Father & The Lost Legend of Pear Tree – Part Two*)

But what of all those who cannot see a way out, who are not able to communicate their thoughts or feelings, have no energy to engage, no ability to seek help? How do we help them? Anxiety and depression sap their spirit. Suicide will amputate it. Secrets can destroy lives. Especially the lives of those who try to convince the world and themselves that they are not suffering. These people need to know there is no need to hide and that there is a way out if they seek to destroy the stigma of mental illness. There are agencies out there that they can talk to who will understand what they are going through. You are not alone. It's time that our community stopped ignoring the most vulnerable that are obviously in need of help. We need to accept that mental illness corrupts the mind. Let us all take the onus if we see someone in difficulty. We cannot leave it in the hands of those who suffer. We need to show them the light. Help is out there; if only we can help them to access it.

For too long, the Punjabi community has treated mental health issues as a taboo subject. This has resulted in many within our community not being in a position to adequately help all those that experience mental health problems. This stigma needs to be eradicated and confronted head-on by us all. Enough is enough; too many lives have already been destroyed, and continue to be devastated by not dealing with the issue appropriately and effectively. Let's be honest, we all know what mental illness is and the debilitating effects it has on those who experience it. Even though we don't have a word for it in Punjabi, we are all aware of how it makes people behave and feel. Our greatest problem, therefore, is not that we don't have a specific word for depression, but that we don't talk enough about mental illness within our everyday lives.

As a community, many Punjabis follow the Sikh faith. One of the fundamental outlooks in Sikhi is the feeling of always being in a positive mind. The notion of Charhdi Kala 'high rising spirits' – the Punjabi term to aspire to maintain a mental state of eternal optimism and joy. Now, this is a wonderful outlook on life if you are in good health, but it is impossible to accept and live this way if you are going through a serious mental health crisis. Charhdi Kala and prayers alone will not raise the spirits of someone who has found themselves consumed by the darkness of a mental breakdown.

In addition to this, anyone who decides to share their inability to live in Charhdi Kala with others may themselves become ostracised by the people they confide in as well as the wider community when news leaks out. Many of our own people do not want to be associated with such a negative attitude to life. Some even say that if you can't follow the path of Charhdi Kala, you are not a true Sikh.

Yet, it is the corruption of the mind that makes someone feel so low and dispirited, not a personal choice. In my life, I have come across numerous mental health disorders within our community: anxiety and panic disorders, bipolar disorder, dementia, depression, schizophrenia, and so on. Each of these is caused by a mixture of biological, psychological, and environmental factors. For example, people who have a family history of mental health disorders may also be more prone to developing one at some point during their lives. Psychological factors and environmental factors, such as upbringing and social exposure, can form the foundations for harmful thought patterns associated with mental disorders. Changes in brain chemistry from substance abuse or changes in diet can also cause mental disorders.

The consumption of alcohol within Punjabi culture is a factor contributing to the dual diagnosis of a mental illness and a comorbid substance-abuse problem. Punjabi culture has accepted the consumption of alcohol to be a norm; it has been the perceived norm since the mass migration of Indians after the Second World War. This drink culture has been passed down generations without our community ever truly understanding or accepting the immense harm it does to us all, and especially to those with mental health disorders. This is fundamentally a problem of culture and not Sikhi in general.

Sikhi alone is not going to provide us all with the cure that certain members of our community desperately require. This is not to say we must abandon Sikhi when seeking assistance from mental health professionals. Religious practice can still be integrated with medical expertise, but pursuing a religious lifestyle in the hope that Sikhi alone will cure a mental disorder is an approach that religious leaders must not continue to promote. With this approach, I believe we will continue to abandon those that experience the most extreme disorders, by pushing them further into isolation. People with mental health problems need expert medical advice and attention, not to be shut away and trapped in their own thoughts.

I know that there are Sikh organisations that combat the issues our community faces regarding mental health issues, and I'm quite sure there are organisations out there that are catering to the Punjabi community, but more needs to be done. Our community needs to steer vulnerable people in the right direction. People with mental health problems and their loved ones need to be provided with information and support from within the gurdwaras and community centres.

Our people are renowned for their strong spirit in times of crisis and adversity. We must now learn to help those among us whose spirits have been broken by the effects of mental illness. We must engage in conversation with all those that have problems and let it be known to them that they are not alone, that we will stand with them, and fight for them. For, is that not the Sikh way?

Let us keep talking. Keep moving on. Keep the faith. Let us disown the stigma of suicide within our community.

Dear Friend with the Old Friend

Eljae

(for Y)

you welcomed death in when it came to your door – spoke
of it like an old friend you'd not seen in a while. you ushered
in, offered a seat, then tea to this figure; rested easy in the
knowledge that soon it would be over. instead came the terror:
knowing how simply you'd let this all go. and now, you tell me,
you're left with a belly emptied by the friend who ate you out of
house and soul; a rapt mind consumed by truth-seeking.

finding purpose isn't easy, I know. been a while since we've
met, I know. still, you are doing the hardest thing: seeking to
survive yourself. and the fight? brutal. nauseating. exhausting. I
know. each clutch weakened by atrophy and surrender, each claw
barbwired by burden. now, finding sweet relief in an end not
your own? seductive, *I know.*

if this isn't bravery, nothing is.

your friend, always,
el

Highlights

Becky Balfourth

On my last night, I accepted a half-lit fag from Racist Scottish Woman. She'd let it burn and burn until it was as much ash as unspoiled tobacco, but I flicked the cherry and took a draw. 'We'll share it,' she said. It felt like an ending, a soap, or a sitcom, or *Girl Interrupted* drawing to a disappointing climax. I saw Smurf, Dora, and Old John watching from inside, laughing, wondering how I'd got that desperate for a fag. Doesn't smoke, Smurfy mouthed in a way that made it clear the end of his sentence would've been: my arse. But it wasn't that. I'd decided that five minutes of listening to the potential efficacy of the pterodactyl as an alternative to the Flying Scotsman was better than going back inside to be watched. She slipped me the end of the fag and went inside. I opened the door for her, balancing one-handed so as not to contravene smoking laws (IT IS ILLEGAL TO SMOKE ON A MENTAL HEALTH UNIT, the door sign and the nearby nurse's face said).

You know what? I didn't use to smoke. Really. Since the age of fourteen, I'd had about five fags in my life. But the mental health unit that January was like a pub just after the smoking ban. All the socials happened outside. It was cold out, and it was an acquired taste, like olives, but it helped. I brushed my teeth six times a day, then soaped up to the elbows every time I was done. Penance, or maybe an attempt to hide the signs in case my family came to visit.

When they did, the faint smell of smoke I was convinced lingered in my hair was the least of anyone's concerns.

Inexpert and shaky at first, I got others to roll for me. Sunglasses sat about making jokes about sucking deep or kissing the box-lighter affixed to the wall. The first puff was always a highlight, like popping the menthol bit on a new Pall Mall. Highlights, bear in mind, weren't all that exciting in that place. Highlights included wiping misplaced apostrophes off the lunch menu, or better, changing them to rude words, though this was more the domain of Sunglasses. Highlights included being permitted to use your own phone charger, unsupervised.

Days were different colours. Yellow and greenish-black pills at a.m. and p.m. and p.m. again; four 'smile Ingrids' (I called them this because they reminded me of a colour I once saw on a B&Q colour chart) twice a day; flat white tablets to make us treacly at night, sweet, thickened, softer, hard-pushed to try running. In between, fags, fags, fags. I measured my steadiness by them, learning to smoke without missing my lips. Suck, hold, and exhale. The courtyard is where Smurfy let me cry on his shirt and promised me it would get easier, and I believed him until I went back inside and remembered where we really were. It was my first admission for a long time, and at that point, trudging frost back into the lounge, I felt people like us never change. It's something I heard a nurse say once. I tried to shake it at the time, but clearly, it stuck. We do not change. And though I liked him, Smurfy's history (alcohol–hospital–alcohol–prison–alcohol) didn't do a lot to change my mind on that score.

The courtyard is also where Racist Scottish Woman called me a 'Paki fucking doctor'. I was incensed; I threw a wet facecloth, a book, a mislaid punch, and once, days later, a snowball at her back. Soon after, she informed me that she loved 'my people' and our 'beautiful silk saris'. I told her to get one of her own and change out of her pissy sequined skirt. It's one of the words I hate most. Actually, I'm Dutch/Irish/Jamaican, and it also upset me that people like her always lump 'people like us' into one category and insult us accordingly. Smurfy told me not to get wound up by her, but the snowball made his day, I could tell. I felt bad about it later and used the boiling water, stupidly placed, meant for tea, to burn my arm. I hid the long red mark, and a week later, it was infected. I felt this was some kind of karma. I didn't know why I should apologise to a racist, but the urge to do so was strong – probably because she was so unwell. The nurses told me that. 'She's unwell, don't mind her.' They wrote in my notes, I later found out, 'inappropriate anger'.

'Fuck Off,' shouted Old John as we walked in after the snow-ball. It was his favourite phrase. 'You old fucking boot,' he shouted at Racist Scottish Woman, then tipped his hat at me and winked in a kindly, rather than a pervy, sort of way. The 'Fuck Offs' were often aimed at me too, but I was taught to respect my elders, and this man was ancient. People thought he had been there, on the allegedly acute unit, for a million years. As well as the swearing, he did save me occasional winks and also kept one of my mislaid socks in his jacket pocket for two days and returned it to me. This got rudely reflected upon by Sunglasses.

Sunglasses swore he wasn't a hipster or whatever but had some kind of light sensitivity. I 60/40 believed him. Rude reflections were his main domain. He gatecrashed games of Scrabble in the Quiet Room to reveal the potential of any word to have a sexual meaning and/or to examine my tits. I was one of only three women, and one, Rachel, when not in her room crying, was still swollen-breasted from the baby she'd recently given birth to. I rarely saw her except at dinner, when she ate two plates a night, one arm held around her stomach while the other shovelled in the food.

Sunglasses brought in his guitar once. 'If your music brings the tone down as much as your conversation,' I said, 'I'd rather not hear it.' It was one of my quicker, between-med, post-smoke moments. I felt a bit bad, mean, 'til he laughed and rolled me one for a mid-game break and everyone laughed at me for 'Not Smoking' as I knelt by the wall-lighter and waited for it to take. (Sunglasses: You do spend a lot of time sucking boxes.)

Lowlights: nights. Sending texts, slow through treacle and bad signal, losing friends in 160 characters (I had a rubbish phone, so after 160 characters, it turned into a whole new message. But usually, it only took one line to screw things up.) The day I left, I forgot my phone between the bed frame and mattress. The hospital never called, so I never collected it. This means I have no record, mental or digital, of what I said to people. All I know is that I had friends when I went in and, when I came out, I had none.

My roommate, Dora, snored. No pills, no iPod, no dream could block out that noise. Sometimes, I thought she had stopped breathing; her snores would catch, and everything would go quiet, and somehow that was even worse. Would it be my fault if she died? Should I call a nurse?

Highlight: at least she had a way of getting them to sneak her out at five in the morning to smoke a sleep-fag and give me a draw. Which I 'Didn't Smoke'. It was her sixth time in that place since last January, so she knew how to get around rules. No one resented her for it; she deserved some flexibility after all she'd been through. When she came in, she had bruises on her face and upper arms, and it occurred to me, talking to her days later, that the person who caused them was walking around free while she and I were making bracelets out of painted macaroni and trying not to cry. Yet, she always highlighted the bright side for everyone else, knew how to make us lost souls feel special.

Dora used to sing in a high, clear, beautiful voice. Almost always religious songs. Once she sat me down and asked if she could sing for me. I said yes, but the whole thing was very intense and uncomfortable as she gripped my hands and talked about how the music would save my soul, so the next time I suggested a fag instead. I admired her faith, but didn't want to be infected by it. I was amazed, with the amount she smoked, that she could hold a note.

I wasn't a total bum; I did once buy a pack for everyone when I was finally allowed, supervised, over the road to Tesco. The nurse pretended they were for her when I got ID'd. It was nice of her; there was no need for her to do it, and she could have gotten herself into trouble. Walking out of the shop, I felt emboldened, triumphant with the purchase of my First Pack of Fags, a twenty-pack of Marlboro Gold, wanting to share them so that everyone knew I had something to give as well as take. Unfortunately, that was also the one day I could be bothered to wash my clothes, and I left the Marlboros in my pocket, unused to the idea of caring for them. I pulled out some matted paper and heavy, gummed-up tobacco from the back pocket a few hours later, after a long search and my unfounded, and thankfully unvoiced, accusations of theft. Lowlight.

The day Dora left, she sparked up a fag in the lounge. 'I don't fucking care anymore,' she cried as one of the healthcare assistants prised it from her fingers. 'What does it matter? I'm gonna die anyway.' To pay them their dues, they were kind to her. They sat and talked with her for a long time, but it must not have helped because when I went to say bye to her, she was zoned-out and droopy. I wished there was something I could do, but I knew that even if I gave her my number, we would never see each other in the Real World Out There; it was not that kind of place.

The next night, my final night, my final highlight, standing

alone in the courtyard and crushing underfoot the last of that cigarette as it started to rain. I lifted up my face, wiped the droplets
off cinematically and realised with a sense of calm and self-
satisfaction that I forgave Racist Scottish Woman. I knew that, in
the morning, I would not say proper goodbyes, so I waved good-
night and promised I'd be good – or at least careful – when I left.

To Braise the Belly Right

Minying Huang

1.   Recognise the ache in your belly.
       Be gentle with each cut. Take a

2.   hot bath: strip down, float starfish
       among the bubbles; soak; ooze

3.   oil. Slip-step from rock to rock over
       low heat. Sweet rock melts against

4.   skin, which turns caramel (giddy with
       flame underfoot and running over

5.   in haste), somersaults and strokes the
       sides of the pan and my heart, stokes

6.   desire for touch and taste. Dark soy
       pops beneath lids – lean in close to

7.   catch fragrance when they fly open.
       Shyly, read the sundial. Reach, blasé,

8.   for wine called yellow fermented from
       rice. Gaze at stars flung from space

9.   into pools around your ankles and your
       waist, smouldering with ginger glint

10.   and hint of spice. Let sugar snow-fall,
       dust your arms of gold. Soften more,

11.   cling, wrap yourself tender around
       fork lifting you far away from here

12.   where it hurts, it hurts. Cradle: your
       bàba's eyes, your māma's eyes.

. . .

20.   Sing when sting comes close. Not a
       promise of protection but of
       the holding of a hand.

. . .

n.   Recognise the ache in your belly.
       You bring joy. You bring joy.

Postscript

It feels odd to be revisiting this poem in 2021, over three years later – not odd as in bad, but odd as in: I'm not quite sure how to feel. So much has happened since then, yet much of what I was going through feels familiar, even now. There was so much I didn't understand about myself; there are many threads tying me to the voice speaking the poem.

In a way, I think *The Colour of Madness* marked a beginning after a beginning. Reading and being a part of it opened me up and gave me permission (not that we need permission, but it helps when you have little to no access to images of possibility) to acknowledge that I was having a difficult time, that what I had experienced and was experiencing wasn't necessarily typical, and that maybe I didn't have to attribute that difficulty to personal deficiency. For the longest time, for reasons I am still uncovering in the present, I felt that I didn't have permission to not be okay.

When I finally sought counselling after a nervous breakdown following a triggering incident, first through my university and later through the NHS, I really struggled with the word 'trauma', which others were using to describe my experiences, including childhood experiences suddenly thrown into a harsh new light. It felt too heavy, and I felt undeserving of it. I still hesitate to use the word. I am still struggling in the unlearning, but I am trying. And I think the speaker of the poem was trying, as if to say: I want you to know, 'You bring joy, you bring joy.' I want them to know that they did, that they do. And I want you to know that you did, you do.

Green

There are times we see in green. Winding vines, intertwined, reaching.

Invisible Shorts

Diljeet Kaur Bhachu

Talking:
My family knows how to talk.
We talk a lot.
But we don't know how to *talk*.

Aunty Spy:
Chk chk chk. The women gossip. I can hear them. In my
  head.

Nobody cares about me,
I'll die and you'll just leave me in a ditch.
I'll die here in the kitchen and no one will notice.
        – a letter from Brown mum.

We'll see. Maybe.
        – a letter from Brown dad.

An ode to meds:
Citalopram, my friend.
On you I can depend.
Until the bitter end.

The Long Goodbye

Olorunfemi Ifepade Fagunwa

I remember the day I arrived at the Spilfest Eating Disorders Unit; we all just stood there staring, our eyes circling, scanning how bilious the room looked. Two beds with white sheets, baby-blue walls, and white wooden side cabinets that looked like they had come right out of an Ikea catalogue. The nurse who had seen us on arrival appeared confused by the presence of our family in such a place, not that I blamed her. She had already directed us to the Pentecostal church three miles down the road before finally checking her list of new patients, and there I was, third from the top: Foyinsola Oluwatimileyin Ademolake.

Once I was in what would become my new room, my mother's need to gain control over the situation was palpable. She wheeled my travel bag to the bed under the window, inadvertently deciding where I would sleep. She opened the pale wooden cupboard, the only thing in the room that remotely stood out, and ran her fingers across the bottom shelf, the dust rolling onto it. She held her index finger out, observing her now-contaminated skin. 'One of you, pass me the white cloth; it's in the small bag,' she said, still maintaining the hybrid Nigerian-English accent that she had used to speak with the nurse. Mide was carrying the bag in his hands. He rummaged through it and brought out the pack of white cloths, passing them to Mother.

'I asked for one,' she snapped. Mide creased his face, looking at me out of the corner of his eye, the way he always did when he had something to say that couldn't be said out loud. He threw the bag on the bed, opened the pack, and handed one cloth over to Mother. Mide creased his nose at her again. *She didn't even say thank you,* his eyes said. She wiped down the cupboard muttering to herself in Yoruba about the many diseases that one could catch from the dust that lay within it.

Unconvinced by the cleanliness of the cupboard, she walked across the room to the sink, opened the tap, and ran water over the cloth. As she rinsed it out, she caught a glimpse of herself in the mirror sitting above it. In that moment, I could see the disappointment, the fear, the exhaustion in her slightly puffy eyes, and she could see it too. I wanted to tell her it wasn't her fault, but it was too late. I had forced her hand, and now someone else had to look after me. She took this as a sign of having failed me somehow, and no matter what I said, she would always believe that this was the case.

Having somewhat satisfied herself that the cloth was now clean enough to use, she turned off the tap and continued to wipe down the cupboard, this time with even more force as she mumbled what sounded like a prayer. She pleaded the blood of Jesus and bound evil spirits, while remembering to rebuke and reject them along the way. The cupboard began to shake, becoming increasingly unstable on its feet; it was as if the spirits had heard her and come to life. Once content, she began to unpack my bags, hanging up dresses and jumpers, folding trousers and T-shirts, placing them where she felt it would be easiest for me to access them.

Mide and I sat side by side on the bed, looking at our phones, texting each other; the room did not allow for conversation.

Do you think she'll ever leave?

No

Do u think she'll b moving in here?

LMAO. I hope so.

Not funny. Make sur u call me b4 u sleep 2nyt.

Defo. Promise.

Mide lightly jabbed me with his elbow; it had felt quite sharp against my skin, but most things did.

'I guess we should be going.'

I couldn't believe my ears; she was actually ready to leave. My mother, who was a procrastinator when it came to leaving for anywhere. She had to wake up an hour and a half before work because it took her an hour to get ready and another half an hour to leave. I felt a slight resentment towards her. She had never known how to be quick about anything, but had chosen today to learn.

My father, who had not spoken since our arrival, had been sitting on the unoccupied bed across the room from us reading his week-old *Punch* newspaper. He rose to his feet, leaning on his knees to support himself as he stood up. He was a tall man, sturdily built with a small gut protruding over his trouser waistband, which he often described as a sign of 'good living'.

'Are we ready?' he asked.

'We're ready,' Mother replied.

'Shall we pray?'

We came together and held hands as my father's heavy baritone voice took 'Blessed Assurance' as our pre-prayer hymn. My mother sang off-key, my father sang low and deep, Mide held the melody, his voice far surpassing our choir leader's, and I struggled to get each word out, fighting back the tears that were trying to force their way to the surface. As my father began to pray, he did not pray with the zeal my mother had exhibited while cleaning; he did not bend to the amateur dramatics that some of the pastors at our church used. He simply prayed for God to make me better, for Him to take away my trouble, for Him to return me to them with a healthy spirit and a full appetite. Together we said the grace, he hugged me tight, kissed the top of my head as I whispered, 'Don't leave me here, please. Daddy, please.'

I could not see his eyes and, therefore, could not see his tears, but I could sense his sadness.

'It is well. You will be well,' he said, and left.

Father and I were close, and I guessed that he, too, had felt the failure one does when your only daughter has chosen sickness over health. He had struggled to understand what this was, and as it grew worse, I felt the need to deny it for his sake. However, it became increasingly apparent from the continuous rejection of mother's jollof rice – the best in the world, I might add – and the stick-like physique that I had adopted over the last few months that something wasn't quite right. Even for a man like my father, my fragile frame could not go ignored.

It had seemed so unlikely that I could be this type of sick. After all, it had been something that belonged only to the Oyinbos. The fact that I walked among them daily, had befriended them, and even looked up to some of them had been of little concern to my father. Inside our house, we spoke Yoruba, curtsied to elders, accepted every young face as our cousin and every old one as aunty and uncle, we argued over Buhari's ineffectiveness and the uselessness of APC and PDP combined, we were thankful for the goodness of God, and snarled at the overly liberal West; we ate amala and pounded yam, recited poetry by Gabriel Okara, listened to Ebenezer Obey, discussed Fela's political incorrectness, played Wizkid jams, shokied to Bobo, while scheduling when we would watch *Lekki Wives*. This was our Nigeria, the one Father created, the one he tried to preserve for us, the one he had hoped would determine our paths. I had fallen off this path; I walked among the outside world. Somehow, I had been given this sickness of the Oyinbos, but he could not understand how.

My mother hugged me as well, and I could hear her choking up as she did so.

'Please, try and eat, okay? The sooner you start eating, the better.' Her Nigerian accent was no longer muddied by her English one.

'I will try,' I replied, hoping that my words would provide her with the strength not to cry. She began to plead and pray, as a rising tide of tears grew in her eyes.

'Please, don't, Mummy,' I said. 'I promise I will try. Okay? Please, don't cry.'

I wiped her tears away with the palms of my hands, and she smiled and hugged me again.

'Mo fi Olorun ṣo e, I love you.'

'I love you too, Mummy.'

'Okay. Bye. Be good,' she said as she walked away, waving with every step.

Finally, Mide and I were alone. We could talk, be free, laugh at Mother's theatrics and Father's disinterest, but we didn't. Mide was my older brother, and even I could see the concern in his eyes as he stepped forward to say his own goodbye.

'Will you be okay?'

'With all the binding, loosing, and the rebuking of spirits Mummy did to the cupboard, I better be.'

Mide smiled.

'I'm surprised she didn't start speaking in tongues.'

'Ah, don't remind her. She might return to finish off the job.' We both laughed.

'Don't leave me here.'

Mide said nothing.

'Didn't you see that nurse? She couldn't even say my name properly.'

'Did you see the side-eye Daddy gave her when she started on our surname?'

We laughed from our souls this time, the weight of the day ever so slightly lifted.

'Are you going to that Skepta gig tonight?'

'Yeah, gave your ticket to Jack.'

The disappointment of hearing Jack would be hanging with Mide over the one artist we didn't argue over was insurmountable.

'Jack? Really? You know I could have come here tomorrow, and does Jack even know the lyrics to a single Skepta track?'

'No. But nobody else was available, and, well, Jack's a beg.'

I folded my arms waiting for Mide to account for his poor choice in companion, but he didn't attempt to bend to my will. I knew deep down inside Jack wasn't a choice that Mide made willingly; Skepta was *our* thing, it wouldn't be the same if we weren't together, but the tickets had already been bought, it was too late to sell them on and besides, he wanted to go.

'Look, I'll send you a video,' he said as he looked at his hands, pulling at his index finger.

'Make sure you call me.'

'I will.'

'Every day. Don't forget.'

'I won't. I promise.'

I hugged him tight, almost winding him. As we stood there hugging, not wanting to let go, not wanting to say goodbye, he whispered, 'Promise me one thing.'

'Anything.'

'Promise me you'll eat. Every day, you'll eat something.'

'I'll try.'

We held each other for a moment longer and then finally, we let go.

He backed out of the room, waving until he disappeared around the corner. I ran out after him, shouting out instructions as to how to deal with Mother as he shouted back that he envied me and maybe he too would stop eating to ensure he wouldn't have to be at home alone for the months before he started university. We did this until we could no longer hear each other and then waved at each other until he became merely a speck in the distance.

I walked back to my room, dragging my feet. I walked past the nurse sitting at the reception desk on the ward.

'What would you like me to call you?' she asked.

'Foyinsola Oluwatimileyin Ademolake.'

She looked blankly at me.

'Foyinsola; that'll do.'

I smiled at her, and she smiled back. I didn't like her smile; it was forced and insincere. I entered my room and closed the door behind me. The lack of bodies in the room added to its sombre tone. I sat on the bed and wished that Mide had stayed longer. I wished that I had asked for him to stay until I had fallen asleep. Instead, I was alone and unwell in a room that was unwell also. Tears filled my eyes, then flooded my face. As I sat down on my bed, I began to pray, and I, too, asked God to help me to eat.

My Baby, Bulimia and Me

Patricia Hope

When you are pregnant and you think about the negative things that could affect your child's health in the future, it is rare that mental health issues spring to mind. At least, this was the case for most mothers-to-be in 1993.

I did all the things that I thought could promote my unborn child's wellbeing. I tried not to become overly stressed, keeping my life and surroundings as calm and positive as possible. I ate a healthy diet and, apart from some prolonged morning sickness, I was in good shape. If you were to ask me if I felt concern over the mental health of my baby, I would have said no. I had not consumed alcohol, coffee, smoked or taken drugs. I had no history of mental health issues in my family. I was aware that my partner's mother was an alcoholic prior to her death, but I can honestly say mental health issues were never a serious consideration.

My daughter was born eight weeks premature by emergency caesarean section after my waters broke early, at which point she was still positioned crossways. As a former midwife, I was all too familiar with the possible complications, but everything happened so quickly. I was in hospital being monitored for back pains and was anaesthetised almost immediately. I did not have time to register anything apart from the potential danger to my baby's life. She spent the first night of her life in the special care baby unit while I recovered on the ward. The first thing the following morning, I was wheeled down to see her with her father. She was tiny, but perfectly formed, and I cannot describe the rush of emotions that swept over me seeing her lying in the incubator with an arm splint and a nasogastric tube. So fragile, yet fighting hard. But somehow, I knew that she was going to be okay.

Fast-forward to age twenty-four and nearly four years of knowing that my daughter is bulimic, I still often look back and reflect on moments in our lives when there might have been signs or warnings that this illness could lay ahead. Research has shown that premature babies are more likely to suffer from anxiety, depression, and other mental health issues; I was already aware that some mothers found it hard to bond with babies that spent time in special care. However, it was not something that I felt was apparent. My partner was diagnosed with depression a few years after the children were born, and as I mentioned previously, his mother had been known to abuse alcohol.

Did any of the above mean that my daughter was somehow genetically destined to suffer from poor mental health, or was it something that we, her parents, had done wrong? Did our move out of London to leafy Buckinghamshire, where she would go to less-multicultural schools, affect her sense of fitting in and subsequently her confidence? Possibly, but we were also surrounded by friends and family from St Vincent (the home of my parents) which we would not have been in London. She also grew up among her cousins as though they were siblings. Did the fact that her brother was born when she was seven and used to life as an only child impact her sense of security and being loved? Did I take my eye off the ball when my mother died and become too lost in my grief to notice hers? Did I overlook its impact at a time she was going through puberty and the growing pains of becoming a teenager? We clashed continually, and our relationship descended into a constant sequence of emotional exchanges and a battle of wills – a total contrast to the relationship I had with my own Caribbean mother, whose word was always unquestionable and final. Did the fact that her father underwent a bout of depression when she was sixteen, temporarily moving out while she was studying for her GCSEs, have a negative impact? At the time, we thought his departure would ease the tension in the house, but in hindsight, perhaps it wasn't for the best.

By the time I became aware that she was suffering from bulimia, it was already well established. It started somewhere between the age of fifteen and sixteen, though it appears she had been binge eating for some years before this. I began to think of all the signs that I had missed prior to her leaving home for university. The food constantly missing from the kitchen cupboards. The all too frequent replacement of toilet rolls (which she used to mask the sound of being sick into the toilet bowl). The need to keep cleaning the underside of the toilet seat from what I thought was urine splashes that seemed not to happen once she left home. The film on the water in the toilet that sometimes didn't flush away after she had used it. The sudden need for fillings, despite her having always had perfectly healthy teeth and cleaning them fastidiously multiple times a day. I could list more, but they all went unnoticed, evident only in retrospect.

Having found out about my daughter's suffering, I had so much to learn and have yet to learn; so many emotions to go through. There is firstly your own guilt that, somehow, you have let your child down or been neglectful in not spotting the signs. Then there is fear, as you learn about the possible consequences of the disorder. There is frustration at the sufferer because you don't really understand anything about the disorder. I remember joking with my daughter at some point in her early teens that I didn't think that there could be many Black people with anorexia because we like our food so much, that it is too much a part of our lives.

Initially, I, like many, thought that the disorder was about appearance and that it was just a matter of accepting what you look like, particularly as every emotion seemed to be expressed in relation to weight, shape and size. It has taken a lot of reading, researching and searching to realise that these are simply a manifestation of the disease and not the disease itself. Bulimia sufferers do not see themselves as others see them and often suffer from other forms of mental illness, such as depression and anxiety. I am told that food, or the control of food, is a way of self-medicating to relieve these feelings, and the sufferer becomes caught up in a cycle of addiction and self-harm. A food abuser (as bulimics are sometimes described) once told me that if you are addicted to drugs or alcohol, you can remove the substance from your life and learn to live without it. Therefore, the hardest thing about certain eating disorders is that you cannot live without your drug, so it sometimes feels like recovery is impossible. Even knowing these things, it is often hard as a parent to be the support that your child needs.

Having supported my daughter for some years now, I would say that the most useful piece of advice I was given was to seek support for myself. Watching your child suffer, no matter how old, can be completely consuming. As Black parents, we do not tend to discuss these things in our community, and sometimes it's hard for someone who is not part of our community to understand why cultural aspects play a role in how we cope and deal with caring for a relative with bulimia. My experience is that many among us are suffering in silence. I have come across grown Black women with their own families who have had and still have bulimia. Sometimes, the biggest help can be hearing someone you can relate to say, 'I know what you are going through because I've been there.'

Sankofa*

Esther Kissiedu

When I was a child, I spoke as a child, I understood as a
child, I thought as a child; but when I became a (wo)man,
I put away childish things.

1 Corinthians 13:11

'You say you are from where?' The customs officer tugged his
tightly curled beard and looked at Grace with the same cool dis-
dain he gave to young kids and street hawkers.

'Abree.'

'ABURI! Pronounce it correctly. You don't look, or sound, like
a Ghanaian!'

Grace hated being corrected, but what she hated more was
being told she wasn't the right kind of Ghanaian.

'I wasn't born here, but I am Ghan—'

'You were not born 'ere, so you cannot claim to be a true
Ghanaian!' He twirled the toothpick in his mouth and made a
suction with the back of his throat.

'I . . . I am,' Grace eventually responded, but it was a beat too
late. He had already stamped her passport and was dismissing her
with one hand.

* Sankofa is an Akan term from Ghana, meaning 'to go back and get it'.

Grace had spent fewer than five minutes on Ghanaian soil, and she had already been chastised. She was used to hearing these kinds of remarks, but this one stung a little deeper – not because of what he had said, but because of her own hesitation – it was the first time that she didn't believe what she was claiming.

As she made her way through Kotoka Airport, she didn't see it at first. It was scribbled in an almost unrecognisable way, as if the concept of writing was fun, but the name was an afterthought. She drew closer to see the words OWUSU, GRACE on a sheet of paper.

'Aah, Grace?' called the short and thick woman who was now waving the name card in Grace's face excitedly.

'Sister . . . Joy!'

'Akwaaba, akwaaba. You are welcome now. Aah, we tenk God you've arrived safely.'

Sister Joy's smile oozed warmth. She was dressed in a green-and-brown camouflage suit, with a matching baseball cap and black working-men's boots, which looked like they were shined several times a day. She was not all how Grace had imagined her. Many summers had passed since Grace last travelled the roads of Ghana on her own, so safe passage through the airport and beyond had been arranged in the form of Sister Joy. She'd thought the whole thing unnecessary at first, but seeing Sister Joy's round, beaming face greeting her, she felt relieved.

'I've been waiting for some time now,' Sister Joy exclaimed.

'Kafra, the flight was delayed!'

'No need to be sorry, you are 'ere now. Woadidi?'

'Yes, I had some rice and fish on the plane, I'm fine.'

'Okay, okay. Mepa wo kyɛw . . . please, let me take dis for you? My driver is waiting for us.'

Before Grace could answer, Sister Joy relieved her of her luggage and happily pulled it into the afternoon sun. Grace stepped outside and inhaled Accra. The sweet-smelling air filled her nose, and the heat wrapped around her so tightly, as if all the years she'd been absent were suddenly joining together to welcome her home. She embraced it.

Grace had braced herself for the often-painstaking ride through the backroads of Accra, where miniature mounds of sand made an obstacle course, and led to a headbanging journey for unwitting passengers. On one occasion, the car dipped so far to one side that Grace thought it would tip over, but otherwise, the journey was smooth.

She gazed out of the car window just as they were entering one of her favourite stretches of road. Palm tree after palm tree ushered them into Labadi. She watched as the beach came into focus; the sun dancing on the water as if inviting her to jump in, if only for a little while. How she craved to run into the sea and let it carry her away.

She wanted to forget what she'd been tasked to do and to feel free like the old times, where she would stay on the beach until sunrise, drinking Star beer and regretting not bringing mosquito spray. But it wasn't a holiday – it was much more than that – so for now the beach would remain a glint in the corner of her eye. A mirage.

'Pure water, pure water!'

Grace nodded her head towards the lady weaving in and out of the cars, and within seconds she was by her window. She took two water sachets and dropped a few coins in the woman's hand.

'Ahh! You be a true Ghanaian,' Sister Joy chuckled as Grace handed her one of the sachets.

Grace had forgotten – or more to the point – ignored the fact that as she was a foreigner in her own land, the water would surely play havoc on her body. As she tore at the plastic pouch and allowed the water to fill her mouth, she observed the water lady moving from car to car and marvelled at how she managed to carry everything so well balanced on her head without letting a single thing fall.

* * *

Grace didn't know how long she had been asleep, but the sun was low, and the streets were eerily quiet. 'We are 'ere.' Sister Joy's voice came as a whisper; her bubbly demeanour replaced by solemnity. Her eyes were widened, and her face had softened. She watched Grace intently.

'Driver, wait for us.' She turned back to look at Grace, 'Let's go!'

The road leading up to the building was desolate. It was discreetly located as if deliberately hidden from the world, only known to those who sought it out. Grace made her way to the welcome desk.

'I'm here to see Mr Asa. He's expecting me.'

The receptionist, engrossed in her programme, didn't acknow-ledge Grace but instead hissed at the TV.

'Please, can you get Mr Asa?' Grace repeated with a little more force.

This time she looked up at Grace; she shuffled her weight from side to side before getting up.

'Follow me.'

The receptionist led Grace through a secure glass gate and out to a small community courtyard that was surrounded by a block of rooms. Grace was instructed to wait on the bench. The courtyard was bare, apart from a small strip of brown grass that ran down its centre and two flowerpots adorning either side. In the stillness, Grace suddenly became aware of the pain in her chest that had been building since her plane journey. She took three deep breaths to steady her nerves, and got up to explore the courtyard, ignoring the request of the receptionist.

The place was too quiet. Grace circled the perimeter of the courtyard, peering into each room she passed – they were cramped, each containing three beds with little space between them. She noticed they were vacant of their usual guests and wondered whether they had left of their own accord. At one window Grace paused, noticing in the far corner of the room an elderly woman hunched over, rocking back and forth. Her head was covered with bald patches, with just a few strands of matted grey hair remaining. Her dressing gown draped off her wafer-thin body, making her look as though no one had paid her any attention in months. Grace felt her heart sink. She crossed over to the other side of the courtyard and hurriedly searched the other rooms with a growing sense of urgency.

Several rooms later, Grace saw a woman curled up on a mattress, gently tapping her foot on the end of the bed. Grace's pulse quickened. She edged closer to the bed, still uncertain. It was only when Grace was arm's length away, the woman stirred and turned to face her. At first, a look of confusion spread across her face, and then she smiled, revealing a gap-tooth.

'My daughter, is that you? I told them you were coming, I told them you would come back for me.' Each word felt like a burning stone coursing down Grace's throat, hitting the pit of her stomach with a thud. They sat together in silence just taking each other in. Grace noticed a sadness in her eyes that was never there before – one that was intense and unmoving. Her once-thick black hair was now crowned in a silver glow, and her cheeks were puffier than Grace remembered. She contemplated whether this was the side effect of medication or from her love of food; she could devour a whole chicken in minutes then moments later say she was hungry.

'I've missed you, my daughter.' She shuffled herself off the bed and moved towards the small wardrobe in front of her, gently taking her clothes from the shelves and folding them onto the bed.

'I will pack my things, and then we can go.' She hummed as she organised her belongings, excited at the prospect of finally leaving the dwelling that had held her captive for so long. Grace watched, words failing her and time escaping her.

'I need to get my hair plaited; they won't do it for me here.'

'I'll do it for you,' Grace finally said, as she watched her intently, sadness welling up inside.

'No! We'll do it when we get outside. I don't need to spend any more time here.'

'We have time; let me plait it for you.'

She eyed Grace with uncertainty and desperation, her hand grasping the bag, ready to leave. Grace averted her eyes, unable to hold her gaze. She released the grip on the bag and said, 'Okay.' Grace reached for the comb on the side table, and as she angled it towards the woman's hair, the memories of long ago came flooding back. It used to be Grace sitting on the floor with her head between the woman's knees, her hair being pulled back as she winced in pain. She longed for those simple times. But those simple times were long gone.

The light outside was fading, and Grace knew her time with her was coming to an end. Mr Asa would be waiting for her. She finished off the last plait and brought her face to hers. She looked regal. Grace smiled, and the smile was returned with a small chuckle, her eyes dancing in the sunlight. And just then, Grace caught it – for a small moment, she glimpsed her mother. The person she knew when she was a child, before everything changed. Grace pulled her up from the floor, and as she did, her arms tightened around her, not wanting to let go. Her mother let go first and moved over to the bed, returning to the foetal position that Grace had found her in.

'I'm going to find Mr Asa,' Grace said. Her mother resumed her humming.

'I love you.' The words rang into the air.

Grace stepped back into the courtyard and released the tears that she had held in for so long. Mr Asa was waiting for her at reception along with Sister Joy.

'Are you ready?' he asked.

Grace nodded. He handed her a round small vase; it was black with gold writing on it. The letters gleamed: IN MEMORY OF A LOVING MOTHER, DAUGHTER, AND FRIEND. Grace turned around and walked out of the estate. Sister Joy threw her arms around her and pulled her in closely.

As the door closed behind them, Grace noticed a small plaque on the door that had gone unnoticed before.

PRIVATE PSYCHIATRIC CLINIC. ONCE ADMITTED, NO PATIENTS CAN EXIT PAST THIS POINT.

Cover Versions, Cover Stories

Suchandrika Chakrabarti

'We feel the same emotions for our ideas as we do for the real world, which is why we can cry while reading a book, or fall in love with movie stars. Our idea of humanity bewitches us . . .'
Roger Ebert in his review of *Solaris*
(dir. Steven Soderbergh, 2002), a remake of *Solaris* (dir. Andrei Tarkovsky, 1972), based on the 1961 novel of the same name by Stanisław Lem

I was recently asked to choose five songs for an appearance on Soho Radio, a mini 'Desert Island Discs' as the presenter, Nina Davis, puts it. I chose tracks connected to a solo show that I'd written at the end of the last UK lockdown, in May 2021, and had performed at fringe festivals over that summer.

'I Miss Amy Winehouse' is a show about nostalgia, partying and grief, seen through the lens of the late singer's talent, stardom and painfully short life during the 2000s. At that time, I was in my twenties, working and partying in Camden, where she lived and was often spotted on nights out. I'm a fan of her music and always thought I'd bump into her in a pub eventually (I never did). She felt real and nearby in the way that superstars rarely do. In that decade, I was also dealing with the early losses of both of my parents. Unsurprisingly, I was creatively blocked, and I admired how Winehouse could so quickly turn her pain and her heartbreak into art.

For the Soho Radio show, I chose songs connected to the late singer: 'Tears Dry On Their Own' (Amy Winehouse, 2006), 'Ain't No Mountain High Enough' (Marvin Gaye and Tammi Terrell, 1967), 'Killing Me Softly With His Song' (Roberta Flack, 1973), 'I Say a Little Prayer' (Aretha Franklin, 1968) and 'Valerie' (Mark Ronson and Amy Winehouse, 2007).

What these songs have in common is their use of sampling and covering. While the relationships between them are not always immediately apparent to the listeners, they're in the minds of the artists, the writers, the band members who make these connections and transform one song into another. Tracing the history of a sample or cover reveals so much about the creative process.

Winehouse's 'Tears' has an interpolation from 'Ain't No Mountain', which is a sample that is then re-recorded; Aretha's showstopping version of 'Say a Little Prayer', a 1968 song I first heard in the 1990s, exists as a complete contrast to Dionne Warwick's smaller, more intimate original; and 'Valerie' is a cover of The Zutons' 2006 song that did so well, the lead singer of the band bought a house with the royalties in 2008.

The most meaningful of these tracks to me is a cover that most of us have forgotten is a cover: 'Killing Me Softly With His Song' by Roberta Flack. She first heard the original by Lori Lieberman in the year it was released, 1972. It had failed to chart, but Flack's version went on to spend five weeks at number one in the American charts. The song brought Flack huge success, including two Grammy Awards in 1973 for Record of the Year and Best Female Pop Vocal Performance. In 1996, The Fugees covered 'Killing Me Softly'; the song topped the charts in over twenty countries, including the UK, where it remains one of the fifty bestselling singles of all time in the UK. The song also samples a sample from the 1990 song 'Bonita Applebum' by A Tribe Called Quest, who had sampled the riff from the song 'Memory Band' by Rotary Connection.

I knew nothing about any of this when I first heard Lauryn Hill of The Fugees singing their version on the radio when I was thirteen. I just really liked the song. Then my mum came into the room and a faraway look settled on her face as she smiled and said, 'Oh, there's that Roberta Flack song.' For her, the years between 1996 and 1973 gently collapsed, and the music took her back to another time. It was a time before me, before she was married, perhaps even before she had ever left India. The song spoke to her in a way it couldn't to me at that moment, the internet not having entered our lives yet to let me search for it. I was used to this feeling of having missed out on so much of my parents' lives and having to learn about them backwards. Their vinyl records, piled up in the corner of the dining room, were as obsolete as their Indian passports by the time I was born in 1983. I caught up on their past through the stories they told me.

It would be years before I would hear Roberta Flack's version. Until then, all I could do was imagine my mother's experience, the moments she associated with that song, the source of the mysterious smile on her lips. I liked to think of her experiencing joy in her earlier life. I wanted to believe that she'd once had a happy, carefree time before the illness began.

My mum died in January 2000, when I was sixteen, from complications arising from her treatment for schizophrenia. When I went back to school a week later, my cover story was that she had died of blood poisoning, which wasn't untrue, but omitted much of the truth. Her condition had deteriorated during my teenage years: she stopped working at a job she loved and withdrew from the world, becoming ever more afraid of the stories that she heard from voices that only existed in her head.

According to my dad, a doctor whose helplessness in the face of her condition led him to become a detective attempting to solve the complex crimes committed against her by schizophrenia, she probably developed it in her teens or early twenties. He feared that a diagnosis would lead to the breakdown of our family, and he was right. She was diagnosed at fifty, then died only two years later; then he died of cancer, aged sixty-one, when I was nineteen, in April 2003. Since then, I have learned how to exist outside of a family unit.

When people are no longer present, they become stories. Decades after her death, I am still trying to analyse my mum's illness for meaning. What was it like to be inside her head? Where did she go during her moments of psychosis? How did her illness shape me? After a psychotic episode ended, she would ask me why I was crying. Did she not remember that she was the reason?

My mum never developed any insight into her condition, never got to the point where she admitted that she had schizophrenia, never accepted that her enforced spells in a mental health unit were to help her. While the symptoms wound down as she was treated with ever more intensive anti-psychotic medications, so too did her joy, her energy, the parameters of her world. The medication left her with tremors. One day she asked me to brush her hair for her, and I could feel between my fingers how much it had thinned in such a short period of time.

Unbeknown to us, she had been refusing the mandatory blood tests required for patients on clozapine (a drug used for treatment-resistant schizophrenia) because one of the rare side effects is drug-induced agranulocytosis, a life-threatening blood disorder. It happens when the body doesn't make enough of a white blood cell called neutrophils. The condition occurs in about one in a hundred patients taking clozapine and has a similar effect upon the immune system that chemotherapy does: it depletes the body's defences against infection. Agranulocytosis is more common in women, and it is more than twice as frequent in Asians as in the white population. My mother ticked both those demographic boxes. Yet, her paranoia seemingly won out over the medical care she should have received. Without the blood tests, the warning signs were missed, and she died suddenly in the night.

I spent much of my adolescent life not telling this one incredibly important true story about me, about our family: not just that my mum had schizophrenia, but that it was the main organising factor of our household. Everything hinged on how well she was, on how soon that unsettling electrical charge would turn up again to poison the air and remind us that she had access to another plane of reality where we could not follow her. It was a terrifying place that left her scared, sad and paranoid when she returned to us.

After both of my parents had died, I gave myself the time I needed to put my mum's story – our family secret – out into the world. I took nearly two decades to do it. The piece was published on the gal-dem website as 'Growing up with a schizophrenic mother: doctors, detainment, and dealing with her death', and it prompted dozens of messages from people who had known me throughout my life. 'We could never have guessed,' they told me. Well, that was the point. We hid it to protect her, to protect ourselves. The word 'schizophrenia' still scares people. I didn't want them to judge her, or me, or us as a family. It was, and still is, the secret that informs every story I tell about my childhood. It's the minor-key chord from another song that nobody knows is embedded there unless they really do their research. I've always had a cover story.

I've written many personal essays about the grieving process I went through in my twenties, and now the loss of my parents is at the core of my fringe show. There is great power and catharsis in standing up in front of people and telling them that my parents died too soon, in asking if they want to meet them (as characters I reinvent for them) and in sharing a few sweet and funny memories of them. Otherwise, there's no one to tell these stories to. I don't think my parents deserve to disappear just because they got ill and died too soon. Their lives and legacies have meaning in the world even now, and I hope my show proves that.

I've only written about my mum's schizophrenia that one time before this piece. I haven't included her illness in what I say about her in the show because I don't think the audience could take it on top of the strand of grief running throughout. Once the audience is feeling too sorry for you to laugh, you've lost them.

Ultimately, I'm wary of how much space my voice should take up when we speak and write about mental health because, after all, this was her illness, not mine. Like my parents' move halfway across the world from India to England, it happened to them, not me; something that began before I was born. Yes, the after-effects ripple through my life and write themselves under every foundational narrative I have to tell about myself, but it isn't a story that begins with me.

My parents died so long ago that they never heard Amy Winehouse's music. I think they would have liked it, especially my mum. The idea of putting all three of them together in a show came to me when I saw a photo of Amy Winehouse's parents standing alongside her statue in Camden Market when it was unveiled on what would have been her thirty-first birthday in 2014. Instead of a daughter, they had a statue, an incredible tribute to a huge talent, and a piece of metal that would outlast us all. But still, where there should be a beloved person, now there was only a memorial.

I wondered what it was – is – like to grieve in front of the entire world, especially in front of fans mourning their own idea of who Amy Winehouse was. I wondered why those fans – including me – felt as though we had known the singer, and took her sudden death so personally. So many documentaries and books are still coming out about her now, over a decade on from her death, trying to solve the puzzle of her short life.

By adding my personal details to a very public story in writing 'I Miss Amy Winehouse', I hope to have found new meaning, not just for myself, but also for other people. It isn't the full story, and it isn't just my parents' story, but it's enough, for now.

I've found that it's far better to write a new version that contains only some of the original chords than to suffocate slowly under the weight of the cover story.

I Am Living Proof

Jason Paul Grant

I am a child of the eighties. One of my earliest memories is of the police entering my house to section my mother and take her away to hospital. She had been diagnosed with a severe mental health condition, which resulted in multiple hospital admissions throughout my childhood.

I am the oldest of five children, so I had to grow up fast, cooking, cleaning, doing chores, and looking after my siblings. When my mum went into hospital, we were looked after by other family members, or we went into care.

I always thought that mental health problems were something that people brought upon themselves. I thought people were weak and that they should just get on with life. I never understood what mental health was all about, even with the experience of family members. Alongside my mother's diagnosis, I have two sisters with mental health difficulties that cause an enormous strain on family relationships.

I made it through my teenage years thinking that I was one of the lucky ones. I managed to get into university, where I studied media and communications. I was able to navigate the competing demands of academic work and part-time jobs alongside managing a student radio station. I graduated with a 2.1 and won a scholarship to study for a master's degree at the top journalism school in the country. I went on to work as a journalist in the UK and across Europe.

In 2015, I travelled to Brazil, and my world as I knew it took an unexpected turn. I started having this feeling that people were after me. I couldn't go back to my hotel, believing they would find me there. I ended up walking around for days and nights without sleeping, completely convinced that someone was after me. The funny thing now is, looking back, if someone was after me, they would have found me. At the time, I was paranoid and delusional without any insight into what was going on. I ended up getting robbed in the night, got completely lost, and tried to board a flight without my passport.

I eventually started to become cognisant and managed to return to my hotel, collect my belongings, and fly back to the UK. After a good night's sleep, I woke up the next day as if the Brazil experience was just a bad nightmare. Knowing what I know now, I should have asked for help, reached out to my doctor, or visited a hospital. Instead, I thought that it was just a bad travelling experience and that I could forget all about it.

Unfortunately for me, I went travelling again, and my unusual experiences returned. Only this time, I ended up in a psychiatric hospital after singing and dancing in the airport. My family had to fly over to bring me back to the UK, which was a complete shock for my partner. Even with that experience, I was still in denial that I had any mental health challenges. I just thought there was a global conspiracy plotting to control my brain and I had to remain silent, as I never knew who was in on it.

About a month later, I was sectioned in the UK. Once I came back to reality, I realised that my mental health was causing my problems. This realisation came as a huge relief that I had not fallen into the matrix; rather, I needed to take some time out. I came to a level of acceptance where I would engage with the patients and staff and take part in the activities in the hospital. I would do mindfulness, play basketball and badminton, do art classes, and go for afternoon walks. Some patients seemed to need more help than others, which gave me the motivation to work towards my discharge as soon as possible.

When I came out, like most people, I wanted to keep my experience private and move on with my life. I moved to Glasgow to study for a research master's degree and built up a lovely life exploring the Highlands at the weekends. Initially, I thought I had put my mental health experience behind me, but my symptoms started to return when I came back down south.

I needed to understand more about mental health, so I became an Expert by Experience with my local NHS Trust. I got to meet people with similar experiences, which was so validating and meant that I was not alone. I got to sit in on meetings, share my views in focus groups, participate in research, and sit on interview panels. After a year, I decided to return to work, and I secured a job as a mental health community partner for the Department for Work and Pensions (DWP). I worked across fourteen job centres in south London, where I trained over 500 members of staff to understand mental health and know how best to support people.

One of the stark realities of working in those job centres was the amount of people who were out of work due to having mental health conditions. The disparities were glaringly obvious, and not much was being done to address them. So, after my contract at DWP finished, I felt compelled to become a research associate at the University of Manchester, working on a study looking at the ethnic inequality in severe mental illness. Some of the stories that we collected were truly heart-breaking.

Then the global pandemic hit. In that moment, I was scared. I thought that all my hard work would come to an end. Fortunately for me, I found a part-time job working as a peer support worker in an Early Intervention Service, supporting people who were experiencing their first episode of psychosis. It was the same service that I had used in the past, so I was able to share my direct experience with the caseload. I also got a weekly walking group up and running, an online peer support group, and would complete recovery action plans with people.

While attending an online conference, I found the Stability Network and discovered that there were people living and working with mental health conditions all around the world. Being part of the network helped me keep moving forward even with the latest lockdown restrictions, as I knew others were going through similar experiences. An opportunity arose for me to join the board, and I have been working with my colleagues to increase the network over the past year. We now have 270 Stability Leaders and are growing every month.

I am so glad that I discovered people like me during the global pandemic, and I hope to encourage you to join the Stability Network if you live with a mental health condition. I want to encourage others to find meaning and purpose without letting their mental health get in the way.[12]

Matriarchal Dreams

Cece Alexandra

One night, I dreamt I was on a boat, and all of my bloodless-faced friends were dying one by one; I was finding out via social media.

I felt completely alone.
Yet not hollow alone.

The white matriarch who used to torture me in Finchley began to torture me in my nightmares. She stood over me as I sat looking for my People, yelling that she was sick of hearing this 'Damn' song. But *this* time, she *can't* touch me, when before she never wanted to.

In fact, she avoided it.

I know my People are somewhere.
I don't even have to look.

This is a contrast to earlier dreams.

Now, my People and I – we cruise on boats while she watches from a distance, unable to touch me on the calm waters that *I* have created.

Nine months ago, she broke my wings so I couldn't fly.

Six months ago, she was breaking my legs to watch me crawl, just for the fun of it.

In my other dreams, the Black matriarch is manipulative for my affection. Suddenly, she is on my side. Suddenly, to her, I am no longer seized by the demonic afflictions for which she had accused me of opening the door to possession over and over and over again. Even drugs, drink, and dirty one-night stands couldn't drown out her repetitive voices.

But over the years, she grows hateful as I learn to stand alone. She changes her tactics; she takes action and cuts me down in my prime with a knife. It has the desired effect; has me running scared in my dreams and running from sleep in real life. I lie awake in terror, wondering what the pale-faced God I once believed in thinks I have done to deserve parents like this?

At first, when accused, the Black matriarch denies the crime altogether but chases me down to beg my forgiveness – to buy my silence with copper love – then in a cruel twist of fate, she tells the court that it's the knife I put into her hand.

What choice did she have? The courtroom gasps in confoundment while the Black matriarch continues to look on, hollow-faced.

'It was the knife *you* gave me,' she repeats.

My Black mother.
She is stronger.
I came from her womb.

Last night, I dreamt of the Black matriarch again. Out at lunch, she stands awkwardly with a mutual friend as her shield. She insisted upon paying; I insisted she did not. Surrounded by my friends, it is clear that my status has changed: I am the one in control. My money-armoured hand swipes her breast pocket like a blade. With the money in her pocket and my back turned, at first, I think I have won, but she follows me. Her domineering anger will not relent. I have offended her, so she stalks me down the street, even as I walk with my friends.

I awake, but she continues to haunt me in my reality.
Until I remind her that this relationship is on *my* terms. Take heed.

The white matriarch said I was aggressive.
The Black matriarch said I had anger issues.

To the white matriarch, I was just an inconvenience eloquently defending myself and my flock.

To the Black matriarch, I was her broken child, birthed from generational trauma into generational trauma like a feeble calf, quietly growing into a broken adult. Yet, I was to be envied, a glorious butterfly regardless.

But these are the guardians of my mental health, the keys to my brokenness, the codes to my fragmented state of mind.

These are my matriarchal dreams.

Mother

Fahmida Liza Khan

I scribble with my pen but the ink falls from my eyes,
Mother tells me to pray it away.

I should be writing on paper but instead I draw on my skin,
Mother tells me I should not harm what He gave us.

Blood flows through my heart but it bleeds from my arms,
Mother tells me I will go to hell if I do not stop.

'What happened?' Nothing; I just fell down the stairs.
Mother, is it not a sin to tell a lie?

I told somebody once but they said they couldn't save me,
Mother tells me only He, the Merciful, can save me.

My head feels heavy now; it is pulling me to my grave,
Mother tells me it is not for me to decide, only Him.

What if I close my eyes forever? Will it all go away?
Mother tells me to get up and give thanks immediately.

If society found out, they would think I am an abomination,
But, Mother, why does it matter what people think?

'Do not bring shame to the family, we did not raise you to do that.'
Mother, I do not know how to deal with this shame anymore.

'They will laugh at you and they will taunt you. Is that what
    you want?'
Mother, my mind is taunted and my skin, bullied. I don't want it
    anymore.

'Your problem is not real, it is all in your head.'
Mother, the voices in my head are hurting me. Help me, please.

'There are people far worse in this world who are dying for help.'
Mother, maybe I would no longer need any help if I was dying.

Postscript

I wrote this piece when I was initially struggling with my move
to a completely new city for my Ph.D; facing even more adversity and much greater challenges ever since. My struggle caused
a clash in culture between where I came from versus where I
moved to, and neither understood each other. It was academic
struggle versus family expectations. I had to figure out how to
bypass it and 'Mother' was my metaphor for culture/society. I am
now reflecting on how I felt and writing this postscript, finishing
my Ph.D in a pandemic where mental health has become a much
bigger concern.

The pandemic highlighted inequalities faced in society, especially for the working class and ethnic minorities. Therefore,

alongside my Ph.D on tribology impact coatings of offshore energy structures, I joined Covid-19 diagnostics, specialising in bioinformatics, genome sequencing and variant/infection detection methods, progressing to becoming one of the National Scientific Leads in the pandemic.

I also worked for Blue Smile, a non-profit organisation supporting young people's mental health and life chances. There, I worked with clinicians and therapists to figure out a quantitative way to enable neglected voices, especially those of young children, to be heard. My time at Blue Smile highlighted how isolating mental health problems can be for young people, especially for BAME children, leading to a domino effect of trauma into adulthood. I'd like to think that the experiences in this anthology were a big contributing factor to how I could integrate BAME experiences into the statistics. It has also helped me realise that mental health can be tackled from a variety of disciplines. After my experiences, I have become a bigger advocate for BAME visibility in STEM (Science, Technology, Engineering, and Mathematics), a field also known to be an isolating environment that can often contribute to mental ill health and imposter syndrome. So I hope that by continuing to progress in this path, mental health struggles can be made more relatable.

almost linear (1, 2, 3, 4, 5)

indyah

1.

Spring 2014.

At least, I think it is.

I am sat wondering, once again, why these rooms always smell so strange, so clinical.

Different city, different decade, different circle in psychiatric hell; same smell.

* * *

This is my first time seeing a psychiatrist. Still, I'm no stranger to these rooms. I've been around and around the 'Counselling and Psychological Therapies' block a few times; I have discovered plenty of shortcuts and side routes. But I'd never been passed off by my GP as 'too difficult to diagnose' or too 'tricky to medicate' before. It is spring 2014, and I am irritable. It is spring 2014, and I am over all of it: the doctors, the psychs, the odd behaviour that I would later find out were signs of my hypomania, the people everywhere asking all the questions I don't want to answer, the night terrors, simply existing. All of it. Tired. And yet, still couldn't tell you what I had done so far that year.

That spring, I bounce between two extremes. There is no

in-between. At times I am, I feel, I speak too much, too loud, and too fast – no, I won't repeat it because you clearly don't care if you didn't catch everything I was throwing at you the first time, okay? The other times I am slow and sorry. I am the high yellow of the wallpaper that she is sunken and trapped beneath, and anything louder than a whisper feels like it will break me. It has been like this for a while now. It will take everyone a while to notice that something out of the ordinary is occurring because, well, aren't those simply the two default positions for Black women in this country? Don't you know that we're usually all hollering about something on the Angry Black Woman™ soapboxes we apparently inherit from our mothers on our thirteenth birthday? Don't you know that if we're not providing some entertainment, we are left to fade into the background, into the shade, as though they're trying to turn us off like dimmer switches? Nobody notices that the weight is falling from my body at a rate that is only matched by the speedy exit of my inhibitions and cares for my wellbeing. Nobody notices that my need for sleep is diminishing just as quickly as my ability to stay in the present moment and not let my life dissipate away.

The psychiatrist. He sits there, scrutinising me from head to toe. By now, I feel I've developed a special ability to read the minds of these types when they look at me in this way. I'm not liking what I'm reading, and I'm pretty sure he's not liking having to interact with me. He sighs and says 'hmmm' over my question-naire answers like they've given him all the information he could possess. Then he starts to ask his dull, patronising questions. Dull, repetitive, reductive questions. I answer them all as well as possible. I just want to leave. 'I'm having trouble hearing and understanding you.' I begin again, louder this time and clearer. I won't be saying it all a third time.

'Did anyone come here with you today?' He knows that they did. 'Is it okay if I ask your friend to come in here and help you answer the questions?'

I don't know, mate. Is it? My back is up, and now I am scrutinising him.

He tells her (not me, of course), 'I'm not really following what your friend here is saying about the way she's been feeling and what's really been going on.' She reiterates. Everything I said, she says. It is almost verbatim. After all, she only knows because I've told her. He thanks her for 'clearing that all up'. As if by magic, the penny drops, and he can understand my position and my mental health fully and totally. As for my friend and her magical ability to be heard where my voice fell, lonely in an empty forest, she is small and has a friendly face. She is white.

Two weeks later, I'll get a letter that says that because of my 'mood issues' he has put me on antipsychotic medication (with no additional mood stabiliser, might I add – whose man he was exactly? I don't know). He won't tell me what exactly I am being medicated for. He thinks 'the minor details will become much bigger than they actually are for Indyah, and won't be of any help for her'. Read: I'm not telling you what I'm medicating you for because you're too fragile to handle that. I had sat there and told him how I survived an abusive relationship and sexual assault. I sat there and told him that, almost daily, I have dangerous, intrusive thoughts and have to fight off urges to do some real damage to myself. And still, I'm too weak to know what I'm dealing with or how best to deal with it. I bet you're not all that surprised that I didn't take the medication straight away and that I demanded to see someone else.

2.

It should not be this difficult to request a different psychiatrist. In a last attempt at keeping myself together, I acquiesce and begin the course of meds. I was at my wits' end and struggling with not harming myself, drowning in the mental memos that made sure to remind me that I was ungrateful, an annoyance, a huge burden, and generally just a pathetic excuse for a person. (At this point, the hypomania was well and truly drying up into the sandstorm of depression that would eventually knock me for six and then come back for more.)

My depression and suicidal ideation are amplified by these new meds, not dampened. I lose my delusions of grandeur, and I am frightened. I am promised call-backs, emails, appointment letters, something, anything. I get nothing. Nothing.

It isn't until my partner makes an official complaint that anyone seems to remember who I am. After calling nearly every day for three weeks, begging for a call from the crisis team, or from the psychiatrist's assistant, worried that I just might not come home one day, he decides enough is enough, and they hear him.

He is big. He has quite a commanding, deep voice when he's angry. He is white.

3.

January 2015. I am no longer capable of working, or sleeping, no longer very good at eating. My body knows only pain, and I am broke in all the ways I now know are possible. I've been sat on the waiting list for long enough, and now they've got me in a weekly group for young adults with bipolar (at this point, I've finally been allowed the double-edged luxury of a diagnosis). I haven't been home to London to see my family in months, close to a year.

I haven't been hugged by my mother in so long it starts to scar my skin, my heart.

I am the only person of colour in the group, let alone the only Black one. I spend the number of weeks that I'm in attendance soothing everyone else and tending to their needs, all the while feeling so out of touch, drowning in distance and difference. A mammy for the mentally ill, if you will.

My application for financial assistance, for both my mental and physical disabilities, is rejected by the government, and the reality of my situation hits my stomach like that one sip too many of tequila. I am too sick to work but too broke to be sick. There's only one solution to this problem; I have to find a job, go back to work, and fend for myself. There's only one problem with this solution, I have to work during the group sessions. It is a toss-up between staying in group therapy and staying alive. But, is it really a toss-up when one side of the coin means surviving, and the other means . . . well, not?

I tell the group leader with as much notice and consideration as possible, that unfortunately, the way my chips have fallen, I won't be able to see the group through to the end. I wish there were some other way; I am committed to helping myself. I tell her it is a matter of keeping myself safe, surviving, and, thus, sane. I tell her that if I could rearrange I would; that I have done everything in my power to look after myself and provide for myself so that I can have a safe space to heal and recover. She tells me that she doesn't think I'm ready to make the difficult decisions that must be made to make the necessary changes in my life; that I am scared, and I am running away. She tells me I am not ready to face my problems head-on. She tells me that she doesn't think it's a good idea, but that I'm free to do as I see fit. I have a hard time not feeling bad about having my hand forced in this direction. I have a very tricky time pushing the feelings of guilt and being a failure from my peripheries. That's the last I hear from her.

She is patronising, grating on me more and more as the sessions went on. She does not understand me. She does not understand any of us. She is white.

4.

It is 2005. Or maybe it's 2006? I'm fourteen, maybe fifteen. It is fuzzy, but somehow, I can see all the fine details. I can see all the lines I have crossed; I can see all the lines I have carved.

I'm sat, for the first time, in one of those rooms that smelt so strange, so clinical, so other. I'm counting all the ridges in the radiator because I will not look this woman in the eye. She tells me that she doesn't have to share anything with my parents unless she feels I am unsafe. I can almost feel my mother worrying and thinking and worrying from down the stairs. She's still talking, and I've counted all the ridges, so I move on to the squares on the carpet, the tiles on the ceiling, anything, just so I don't have to look her in the eye.

My mother drives me to half of my appointments; I leave school early to go to the other half. I believe my father knows nothing of my appointments, knows nothing of the marks on my skin, because 'it's hard to understand.' In fairness, it is. At least once a fortnight, I sit in this room with its whistling radiator and wonder what I'm doing here. I share more and more as the sessions go by, finally feeling like it's not so bad, and, well, at least she doesn't tell my parents everything I say, right?

Our session is coming to an end. I know this because even without a clock in the room, I am aware of how many seconds have passed. Numbers and order are my thing. Out of nowhere, she says, 'If it's okay with you, I'm going to ask your mum to come up and have a chat with us.' I feel like I make eye contact with her for the very first time.

I know then that things may not be okay with me for a while, actually. Unbeknown to me, I am apparently unsafe. So now, she needs to fill my mother in on some of what we've discussed. The self-harming she thought was a rare thing that I didn't do any longer; she's now aware that's not strictly true. The suicidal ideation and just sheer pain and discomfort I was feeling, well-hidden among teenage angst and sarcasm and buried between the lines of poetry and prose, was suddenly exposed. It was all strewn across the table with its rough edges, laid bare for my mother, and what felt like the world, to see. This humiliation, I somehow knew, would not be the end of this ordeal. No, a few minutes later, she would begin to tell my increasingly distressed and frazzled mother, with that strong furrowed brow of hers, what was to me, at the time, news. 'I think your daughter might have a case of what is known as Obsessive-Compulsive Disorder, and I think it would be a good idea to start her on a small dose of—' I forget which specific medication she had suggested now, some sedative, I'm certain. It didn't matter which one it was anyway because my beautifully British Caribbean mother was having none of it. Mum promptly decided that it wasn't going to do me much good to keep seeing her; the woman who just kept wanting to give me a prescription but didn't seem to have too much else to suggest.

In my adolescent defiance, I felt wronged and robbed of a freedom that I believed was just around the corner, was just about to be mine, and all I had needed was that medicine! For days, I dreamt of a peace that was being withheld from me, a peace from all the noise, delivered in a simple daily pill that would do just that, no more, and no less.

I inwardly raged about not being understood, about being the black sheep in a Black family. I deeply believed my parents were just backwards Jamaican folk that didn't understand modern psychiatry and definitely didn't understand me (try telling that to my Childline-volunteering, paediatric nurse of a mother and see if she doesn't give you, at the very least, one dutty side-eye). The truth of the matter is, I didn't need medication at the time. Looking back with that delicious glaze of hindsight, I didn't need to be medicated. Was I struggling? Undoubtedly. At fourteen or fifteen, in the midst of all the rubbish and nonsense of puberty, were sedatives going to 'fix me', cure me, or even really help me beyond numbing me? Probably not. Not at that time, no. I needed to actually express these emotions.

Knowing what I know now about medication – antidepressants, benzodiazepines, sedatives, antipsychotics, mood stabilisers – I have the uncomfortable realisation that I spent so many months being so angry and upset with the one person who had my best childhood interests at heart, who wanted to save me without stripping me of myself before I ever knew myself. Who wanted to give me a chance to help myself and fought against my fighting to help me see that those parts of me that I was often trying to rub out meant something and had every reason to stick around. She was passionate; she was angry, upset. She was the decider. She is my mother. She is Black.

5.

It is 2018. The early months of the year are still trying to kill me with coldness, and this lack of sun is really not the one. In the winter, I take meds to help keep my moods regulated, because this British Vitamin D deficiency is definitely not the one, either. I talk to my loved ones about my feelings, and they share theirs. My family and I discuss emotions and depression around the dinner table like commonplace matters because that's exactly what they are. My lover checks me on my moods, and I check him on his. I break down only what needs to be understood and rebuilt stronger, and I build only on solid foundations.

I am mentally ill; I am all about working to improve my mental health, building and deconstructing in order to expand my mental wealth. I am strong; I am soft. Fragile, but firm in my beliefs and understandings of myself. I understand myself better than I ever have and thus know how far I have left to go to get to my peace and clarity. I am a multitude of things, some more whole and formative than others. I am an extension of the sun's rays and the rain's drops. I am hurting. I am healing. I am Black.

New Mother

Reba Khatun

Congratulations! Is it a boy?
No, she's all dressed in pink as you can see
Oh what a shame, maybe next time you'll have better luck
No, actually she's all I've ever wanted

How's motherhood? All great, is what I'll hear
Not so good, I feel sad and anxious
Pull your socks up, no need to be glum

She doesn't stop crying
That's motherhood, deal with it
The crying is endless
Babies cry, full stop. What did you expect?
Cuddles and naps, smiles and laughs

Is she walking yet?
No, she's not even one
Oh dear, maybe you should be worried
Actually I wasn't, but now . . .

Is she talking?
A few words. 'Mum' was first

Oh dear. Mine was talking sentences before one
Maybe I should be worried . . .

She hit my son. Is there something wrong with her?
She's only a toddler, navigating her way
She's weird, just like her mum
Leave her be

I thought company and support would be nice
But now I see loneliness can have its upside
I was taught to speak kind or be quiet
Something I'll be sure to teach my child

Reality Check

Raman Mundair

I am many things. I am a writer, artist, and activist. I am a woman of colour. I am a first-generation migrant, a mother of three children. I am a survivor. On the street, I look like I've got it together: I'm high-functioning. I appear confident. But after giving birth, I experienced postnatal depression (PND), which stripped me bare and brought me to my knees.

My experience of operating in a society in which structural racism is inherent is largely absent from any measure of my health and wellbeing. When I present an ailment to a medical professional, it is abstracted from my lived context, and fundamentally, my illness is read as distinct from my experience as a woman of colour. The same is true for my experience of PND.

I feel I must say unequivocally – I Love My Children. I loved them from the moment I knew of their existence, and that love never wavered. But PND irrevocably changed me. Looking back, I now know I suffered from PND after the birth of my eldest child. However, I did not admit it to myself until the birth of my twins five years ago. I am still in recovery from PND, and I will never see things, especially motherhood, in the same light again.

It is a strange and isolating space. It is a place ripe with emotion and fragility and has the potential for personal strength, growth, and power. I was doing 'so well', coping and nurturing the twins and my then-toddler. Everyone was 'thriving', as far as the health visitor and doctor were concerned. When professionals asked after my health, and I said I was exhausted, the usual response was along the lines of, 'Of course you are, you have twins.'

Yes, I was physically exhausted, but I also felt like shit. I felt like I was the worst mum ever but couldn't complain because I was blessed with my beautiful, wondrous children.

For an extended period, I existed in a hell state where my babies would cry for hours. They were unable to latch on, no matter how hard I tried, and unable to digest expressed bottle-fed milk. They were in pain. I found myself feeding non-stop to make up for the milk they threw up to ensure that they gained weight. With my first child, I was able to steal some precious time to sleep and recover, but with the twins, I had no such opportunity. My health visitor didn't take my concerns seriously, and after nine long months, my eldest was finally diagnosed as lactose intolerant. With the twins, I was finally offered a lactose-free formula after six weeks. The stress of all this encouraged PND to take a deeper hold.

When I was unwell, I felt I couldn't raise the alarm because I was worried about what the consequences might be. What would happen if I admitted I wanted to crawl into bed and never wake again? What would happen if I spoke about the incessant intrusive thoughts? My fear that my 'bad mother-ness' would mean that one of my children would die in their sleep, which meant that I had to watch over them as they slept. I would compulsively check on my toddler in the middle of the night, and, as she was a light sleeper, I would often end up waking her up, which, of course, added to my exhausted, frazzled state. All the while, my partner slept without concern, completely unaware of the potential for danger I saw all around.

My deepest fear was I would be punished in some way for

some unspecified bad deed with the death of my family. I was the universal mother, hypervigilant and feeling pain for all children. With both my pregnancies, I gave birth at a time that coincided with major child sex abuse cases being reported in the UK national news. The fear for my children was visceral. Day after day, I was traumatised and unable to switch off the news. I felt I had to listen to the details, the awful facts and testimonies. I had to listen for all children. I couldn't switch it off. Why should I have the luxury to choose not to hear suffering?

I felt similarly about the refugee crisis and found myself weeping and in despair. That in itself made me feel self-loathing – how pathetic to feel despair when I was so privileged. One particular image that will stay with me forever was a report that contained film footage of a mother and child refugee in a holding camp on an Eastern European border. A country where they treated refugees like vermin and held them in camps that reminded me of the camps that probably existed in the same geography during the Second World War.

The footage showed the child hungry, malnourished, making weak cries. The exhausted, hijab-wearing mother rocking her baby numbly, tears streaking her face. I had also been unable to feed my children, despite my best attempts. Mine were prescribed special infant formula, for which I am forever grateful to the NHS – they fed my babies when I couldn't. The pain of knowing your child is hungry and not being able to feed and nurture them. God, the nightmare of that!

Here I am, in the rich northern hemisphere, where colonial history and random acts have led me. I am here because 'they' were there. The refugees are on the move because we were there. Everything is interconnected. There is a growing understanding that the world is now smaller and more connected since having access to the world wide web, yet this understanding doesn't seem to stretch to the world offline. There seems to be a missing empathy link – that the human beings crossing borders in desperate need could easily be me and my children, or you and yours.

The exodus of refugees from Syria to Europe is poignant to me. A few years ago, I was lucky enough to be asked to travel from Scotland to Istanbul as part of the Word Express Literature Project as a writer. I made most of the journey via railway. The route I took, the final leg of which was a train from Thessaloniki to Istanbul, will be the same route that many refugees take in reverse. I think of this often. I know that the intensity of my feelings when I was ill was a reflection of PND, but the actual feeling and concerns are not unfounded. The refugees are real and in dire need. Children are at risk of sexual abuse. PND just magnified these realities, making them huge and impossible to process.

I was aware of what PND was, but did not acknowledge that it was what I was feeling until a year after my twins were born. I think I was waiting for someone else to legitimise my pain, for someone to notice, to acknowledge my distress and exhaustion. It wasn't that I didn't ask for help. I did. I asked my mother to come. She was unavailable. So I continued, got on with the job of raising young children without support or sleep, as do countless other parents.

People are always fascinated by twins, the double impact of arresting cuteness, but, somehow, no one is particularly keen to come and help out. Funny that, eh?

In Indian culture, there is an ideal that a child is raised by the extended family as well as the parents; that grandparents, aunts, and uncles all pitch in. Families in the diaspora rarely experience this. My mother didn't. I didn't. Cultural ideals are whimsy and are just that – ideals. Realities are harder to comprehend. It seems obvious, but it took me by surprise – becoming a mother brought up memories of my mother and my experience of being mothered.

This is something that will present with most new mothers, but if you have a difficult or complex history with a parent, this creates more vulnerability at a time when you feel raw and open. I found myself filled with anxiety and distress as the intensity of PND complicated these feelings further, and I internalised the shame and pain around these memories.

Raising children is undervalued and is seen as solely a woman's job. It is a job with inadequate resources and support structures; a job with no access to human resources. The mother alone is the singular human resource. This is not to say there aren't men raising children alone but here, now, I am talking about women. In the small, constantly eroded space where women are allowed to talk about their experiences, I choose to talk about women, and specifically women of colour. Like my experiences as a woman of colour, PND was just one more thing for me to deal with, process and try to survive.

My reality is that I have experienced the effects of racism from the age of three, the age that I moved to live in the UK. From that tender age, I have been aware of the effects of racism on my parents and its consequent impact on our environment; on me and my siblings. As a child, I didn't have the language to express and quantify the experience of seeing a white woman hurl racist abuse at my father for a mild traffic accident (his car bumper was hit) that he was not responsible for. I saw my father lower his eyes and acquiesce to the woman. Later that day, the full force of my father's anger at being disempowered was physically felt by my mother and me.

At four years old, I was aware that the world was a dangerous place. I vividly remember my mother and I having racist abuse shouted at us and being spat at by a group of white men in a Ford. They crawled beside us as we tried to walk down the road. When we went to cross the road, the car mounted the pavement and backed us into a wall. My mother held onto my small hand the entire time. When I looked up at her face looking for reassurance, I saw her face frozen in fear and tears rolling down her cheeks. I can cite many similar incidents throughout the years, and they all build up a concrete experience of structural racism, which has hummed like white noise throughout my life.

Amani Nuru-Jeter, a social epidemiologist at the University of California, Berkeley, is interested in how the lived and social experience of race turns into racial differences in health. For example, her research found that the fact women of colour experience chronic stress from frequent racist encounters is associated with chronic low-grade inflammation; similar to having a continuous low-grade fever. Nuru-Jeter suggests that this could be a sign that chronic stress from discrimination can dysregulate the body and put someone at a higher risk for a condition like heart disease over time.

I would wager that racialised encounters also impacted my mental health, making me more perceptible to PND. In fact, when I was eventually taken seriously by my GP, blood tests revealed that I had also developed several autoimmune conditions. Autoimmune conditions function on a variety of levels, causing havoc with your health and wellbeing, but something they all have in common is that they raise your body's inflammation markers. In effect, your body is so distressed that it attacks itself. The irony of that, alongside PND, which was undermining my mental health, was not lost on me. How do you tell your invariably white healthcare professional that you believe you are ill because of the stress of living in a racist world? Do you dare to do that knowing how people of colour, especially women of colour, are treated within the mental health system? I have worked as a writer and artist inside hospitals, closed psychiatric units and mental health drop-in spaces. I was therefore well aware of what limited help and possibilities were available to me and how easily they could be detrimental to, rather than supportive of, my wellbeing and recovery.

The options for people of colour with mental health difficulties are severely limited and lacking in vision, understanding, and compassion. When I was a student at university, I went through what I now recognise as depression. I went to see my GP at the university medical practice and found myself in a doctor's office unlike any I have seen before or since. Like the study of an Oxbridge don, it was lined with books and dominated by a large oak desk with a sleepy Labrador nesting underneath. I sat across from her in an uncomfortable chair and explained my low feelings. Within moments, electroconvulsive therapy was on the table as a possibility before counselling or medication had even been explored. I left frightened, ashamed and shocked.

I am now on the fragile yet firm road to recovery. A key factor in that has been my realisation that I needed to diminish my 'mental load', and be more attentive, when possible, to my own needs. This is not easy. I began by writing down all the things I did as a mother and partner within our family. I realised that, despite our self-awareness, my partner and I had cruise-controlled into prescribed gender roles. It isn't just about housework and childcare: we believed we were in a balanced partnership, but there was a mountain of 'invisible' labour that I undertook that my partner was unaware of, for example: thinking about and organising the children's vaccinations, new shoes, play-dates, planning meals and sourcing all household and personal items so that they kept within our family budget. When people came to visit, I was aware when the children were tired and needed to be fed, bathed and put to bed, rather than being the one fully surrendering to and enjoying our guests. They appear small, inconsequential things, but when you add them up, it is a weight of incessant, gnawing responsibilities that add to your exhaustion. You are never 'switched off', and it robs you of your vitality.

Writing down all that I do, even the small things, and sharing it with my partner opened up a useful and healthy conversation. We were able to divide up the mental load so that we both carry an equal share. I am grateful that I am in a position where that can happen. Yes, I am many things. I am multitudes. I am in recovery from PND, and I'm learning to live with several autoimmune illnesses. It is a strange dance that isn't linear.

I am now a few years down the line. My twins are five years old and recently began full-time school, and from this distance, I consider the directions I have taken in motherhood and selfhood. I made a point of finding a good therapist and am happy to say that I am now working with a therapist who understands most of the intersections of my lived experience. More importantly, I understand and have much more compassion for myself. I recognise that I have, for various reasons, been shaped by living as a working-class woman of colour in British society, and I have accrued layered and complex post-traumatic stress. My children's birth stories and my PND are interwoven threads in this.

I had to make some difficult and courageous choices to create a situation that was beneficial for all in my beautiful family, including myself. The more attention I pay to my needs, the better mother and parent I am, the better role model and family member I am.

Of late, I have been reflecting on my own precarious experiences of attachment with my parents and of theirs. I understand now that I am a child of people whose land, sense of self and legacy were torn from them during the partition of Punjab by the British. That my parents were born into that violence and fear. That they carried that with them across the ocean and leaked it into me. That I, then, went on to have my own relationship with precarity, displacement, and the stresses of racism and coloni-alism. That intergenerational trauma is part of me, and that I must be mindful of this in my own parenting. The best way I can manage this is by ensuring a level of consistent self-care. I'm not always moving forward, but I am moving. I set the pace, and when I can, I conjure joy, magic, music and dance.

References

Rae Ellen Bichell, 'Scientists Start To Tease Out the Subtler Ways Racism Hurts Health', *NPR*, November 2017, https://www.npr.org/sections/health-shots/2017/11/11/562623815/scientists-start-to-tease-out-the-subtler-ways-racism-hurts-health

Emma, 'You Should've Asked', *Emma*, May 2017, https://english.emmaclit.com/2017/05/20/you-shouldve-asked/

In Lingala, We Call It Liboma

Christina Fonthes

My grandmother said it the day she found her first daughter, Mosantu, asleep in a stranger's bed after the third day of searching. Barefoot, lips cracked from lack of water. 'A beli liboma'.

Aunty Chantal said it when she took me to Kilburn Market. We bought three aubergines and a brown paper bag of garden eggs. Mad Mary walked past us minding her own damn business. A silver trolley full of black bin liners spilling her secret – a black-and-white photograph of her as a bride in white with a man she had not lain with in too many years. 'A beli liboma'.

Cousin Merveille said it when Mama Pathy, the woman who sewed all of our liputas for weddings – being a woman of the word she always made the skirts longer than we asked – started cleaning the pavement outside of her house with a bucket of soapy water at 3 a.m. every morning. The council had refused to move her; they said she did not have priority. No one but her could see the blood stains from her son's body. 'A beli liboma'.

The barber said it the Saturday I went with Uncle Teddy to get his hair cut. The barber held his clipper up to Uncle Teddy's head when he started recounting the story of his friend who was so unhappy with his marriage that he got up and walked out of the house during an Arsenal match without his keys or his coat and never came back. 'A beli liboma'.

Mama said it on the phone to Aunty Lola when she thought I was asleep. It was two days after I came home. I was lying on the leather sofa in the living room. Mama was watching Nollywood and drinking Miranda. I heard the rustling of the sertraline in the pharmacy bag. 'A beli liboma'.

Bike Dream

Temitope Fisayo

He has a seed stuck in his teeth. It's from a pomegranate and it's in there, deformed and a dull yellow. He can't see it but he can feel it, feel how it sticks out, just so slightly, from the natural ridges of his molars. He runs his tongue along them again. The pattern of bumps and troughs are unique to him, would be random to another person. If he ran his tongue over Will's teeth, or Julia's, he wouldn't know the seed, the interloper, from the native enamel. The more he grinds his teeth the harder the seed protests. It will not be shifted by force.

He is watching the boys and girls in his year as he inspects his mouth. They are unconcerned with his teeth, his pomegranate, or his seed. They are their own marvel. They are dancing in the way adolescents do – not with music, or feet, but with cruelty. They cast aspersions like black hexes. *Faggot!* cries one: five seconds bad luck. *Pussy!* hisses another: and so wilts a budding flower of tenderness.

He hates this dance. But it is a complex hatred. While he loathes the chants, and the fighting, and the banter, he wishes himself a part of it too. He would do anything to be called a gaylord. Or at least, to be called one in a way that meant he wasn't one, not really. At the moment no one says anything to him. Nothing personal, anyway, which is why he can sit with the seed in his teeth, and wonder about Will and Julia, and no one will be any the wiser.

Here is where he makes his mistake. He presumes that a friendship, the kind he is looking for (but doubts, really, that he will ever find), installs within the relevant parties a sort of telepathy. It is a mistake easily forgiven. It looks that way from the outside. As he watches them, with his tongue on the well-chewed seed, he tries to chart the signals. They swirl around the room, a flock of subtle flashes. There is a glance that says *let's steal his bag*. Another that says *let's just fucking punch him!* And they do. And it's funny. And the girls shriek, a bit. It is so bizarre that violence has become currency; stranger still how poor he is. He does not like pain. He does not want them to hurt him like that. He is thankful that they don't. He has learned that there are some people you can just gang up on and beat and it will be hilarious and there are others you cannot. It is probably because he is the only Black boy in his year, and if they were to laugh at him as they pushed him and kicked him it would not look very good, for anyone involved.

After careful and dextrous negotiation with his tongue, he liberates the seed from his teeth. It is a mess of seed coat and embryonic cotyledon and whatever else they showed him in Biology and he swallows it. At some point – and he can't quite remember the details here – some seeds have, like, seven nuclei within them; like seven different plant brains, directing growth, colour, and a sprawling hidden list of things that are important to plants. He only has the one. He only has one faulty human brain, glitched and always filling with sadness, like the hull of a sinking ship. His one brain only directs him to keep breathing, keep the heart beating, and neglects the human list of values and virtues like joy and kindness.

He only has the pomegranate to busy his hands. It is not okay for him to sit there as he is and simply stare, at the table in the back corner of the common room. He did that once, and the teacher on duty, Mrs Raeburn, noticed his eyes, and his hair (a feat, for they never notice the hair).

Mrs Raeburn is a stern and thoroughly lovely Scottish woman who considers all the students of the sixth form to be under her wing. When she asks a question about your home life you do not lie, as you might with other teachers, because she has her own software that alerts her to falsehoods. This is a tale she will tell herself – prompted, it appears, by the untruths themselves. On occasion, she interrupts, does not wait for an answer, as she has smelled the lie before it can be spoken. A prodrome of sorts, for the headache that is tolerating bland small talk. (She wants to protect children, for as long as possible, from the dulling effects of social mores imposed upon them by adults.)

When Mrs Raeburn had seen him, he was not able to dissemble that he had been sleeping well. He was unable to conceal the fishbowl around his head that kept others at bay and filtered all stimuli. She had taken him out of the common room (paraded him like a dead man walking) and spoken to him earnestly. *Anímate!* she had said, the Scottish accent again valiantly defeating the Spanish one (her Spanish A-Level classes boasted high grades, despite this). She had recommended counselling, which he had not gone to.

Once, another student (India Sowerby-Wells, famously born in her parents' ancestral home in Malawi, where she still summers, where she gets 'almost as dark as you!') had been late for Biology because of counselling. And then they had all called her psycho behind her back and to her face and when the teacher obliviously assigned her a presentation on neurotransmitters and psychedelic substances she couldn't handle everyone giggling through the whole thing and she ran out of the class crying, which made it worse.

So instead he has resolved to mimic normality. He has his pomegranates. Beside the little flimsy plastic tub is the black plastic spork, which can be crushed into chips and burned for fuel. And beside the black plastic spork is a novel he is pretending to read, in French, but not for French. If Raeburn asks, he will make noises about going beyond the curriculum. But he would rather she didn't ask. It would not look very good, for anyone involved.

He is still doing his anthropology; he is still looking at them. Here is another glance, one that says *I actually quite like you and I only join in with the others to be close to you, because I know you'll watch, and really, I wish we could leave them and actually just talk, you and me, about something real, about the future.* This last one is Will's. Will does not look at him. Will looks at Julia. Will always looks at Julia, but only for seconds at a time. He has noticed this and assumes Julia has noticed too, because girls know everything, because they are vigilant. He would quite like for Will to look at him. He would quite like for Julia to look at him. He would, ideally, have them together, looking at him, and he, they, in a grand ceremony of mutual acknowledgement. The thing about anthropology is that it requires you to be an outsider.

He likes Will because he is soft. Will really likes Biology and still says that he does, with sincerity. That's important. He will probably go to Cambridge, where they keep animals in the fields and basements, and beam endlessly with fulfilment. When Will talks, there is a shining light that suffuses his eardrums in a kind of healing magic. Will always pronounces his name with an egregious African accent. He does not speak this way for any other word. But he did once look uncomfortable when Matty Sails went on another rant about wasting foreign aid on spearchuckers in Africa. He appreciated that.

He likes Julia because she is good. She is a star of track and field with school records under her belt for high jump and hurdles. She is talented, really talented, has a GB vest and all. She is dedicated and motivated and powered by something deep within, which he hopes she will one day share with him. Julia is half-Korean, and half something else that no one has ever asked her about. Julia doesn't notice him, or decides not to notice him, he thinks, but he is happy for her in theory. It is nice not to be the only one whose parents are from somewhere else. They both, on occasion, make the apologies, wave the hands, and explain that beyond the shores of England lie whole other nations of people.

But Will and Julia are matched in a way he finds quite difficult to unwind. They are earthed together, in their group, in their dance. They have a context. He is a weightless speck.

He will not convince Will or Julia of his love, nor his worth. They will all leave school next year and they will never speak again. He will stop existing to them. This comforts him. His love has been his project since Year Eleven. When he first became this way, the joy of it soon vanished, snuffed out like a weak flame in winter. But what remained was the curiosity and the alienation. Now, he is like a piano with its lid removed and hammers muted: you can press the keys and watch the mechanism go through the motions, but gone is the melody that defines the instrument. Soon, he will have no reason to get out of bed. He imagines he will gather dust, or wake up one day a cockroach, or be turned to bits and burned for fuel.

Of course, his parents will not approve. He has no solution to this problem. So far, he has been everything they have demanded of him: he has his academic achievements, he has his cello grades, he liked tennis. He has applied to read a good subject at university, one that will make them proud.

They did not ask for a deviant (a *bisexual*). And so he stopped being one. Or has planned to stop being one. Or is trying to, but is unsure of what exactly in him to switch off. He fears he is a little bit like a Gordian knot, a huge morass of conflicting fibres. The only solution to the puzzle was to sever it completely. He is not there yet. But he is terrified of arriving there, with the sword, and the boat and the shore, and the sunset.

And he knows, too, that his parents have not asked for a difficult child, and so these sequelae are best resolved privately and quickly. A depressed child, in some ways, is worse than a queer one. The queer children can be said to have found their own twisted path, despite their parents' best efforts. That is understandable: some are destined for sin, and we pity their families who suffer their continued deviances. The depressed child is a product of its environment. They are inherently indictments of the family around them, who look guilty by association and whose methods, goodness, and godliness will be questioned. It does not look very good, for anyone involved.

The lunch break yawns on. Will and Julia and the others are still getting along swimmingly. They are talking about parties and get-togethers and club nights. Slowly, the demand for fake IDs is decreasing. Age spreads over the year group as spring does over England, and, like daffodils opening, boys puff out their chests, and girls hold their heads high. Slowly, they thaw free from yet one more aspect of insecurity. He is not invited to any of it anymore. He used to be, back in Year Ten, when he could go to someone's house and squirm as his friends yelled nigga at him, over and over again, to music (though once, a capella). He had grown tired of that. He had, in fact, penned electronic essays pleading with everyone in his groupchat never to use the word again. He had subsequently been excised from the group, like a thorn from a rose. And indeed, they had called him a prick, to his face, before cutting him off from everything.

The thing about private school is that it manufactures people. It takes their raw materials and warps them, through a looking-glass lens, into something called an 'old boy'. This is quite distinct from being a man, which is what poorer people become. Integral to this process is submitting to order, not to justice. This is why, when, upon reports that he would try to escalate things – tell a teacher, even, he was immediately brought in for a 'private meeting' with the head of year, Mr Knight. Mr Knight accused him of cyberbullying his friends, calling them ridiculous things like 'racist', and really causing them quite a lot of emotional distress. Of course, in that kangaroo court, he could only play his part: *weeping brute who doesn't know his own strength*. He could still act then, as he is acting now, in the back corner of the common room, with his pomegranate, and so escaped further punishment.

Being an 'old boy' is not currently recognised as an affliction, but he is working on changing this. After this next summer, he will have survived the whole thing, and he will note as such on his medical records. He will be like a fish that feeds on plastic – sad and marvellous at the same time.

He thinks a lot about the plastic in the oceans. Plastic was built never to degrade, and so it just lies there in the water. They say one day all the plastic in the water will clump together and form its own country. He is made of plastic, too, and maybe one day he will go back to where he came from like Matty Sails wants him to. Back to his plastic nation in the middle of the ocean, toxic to the nature around it, only good to be turned to chips and burned for fuel.

The bell will go soon and he will have to go to double Biology. It will be another afternoon powered by pomegranate seeds. He has not been having school lunches for a week now. Usually his desire to eat peters out much earlier, as soon as he stops sleeping, but this time it has persisted, albeit in a reduced capacity. He skips breakfast at home. He buys Red Bull from the vending machines at school. He eats pomegranates. When at home he doesn't dare insult his mother's (truly fantastic) cooking, and so under her eye he manages some small-small ẹbà, or rice, or yam. She frowns he is subsisting, but does not have Mrs Raeburn's talents, and so is assured by his insistence that he eats big meals at school.

His mother is a troubled amateur gardener. Try as she might, she cannot get her son to grow as she would like. He is still scrawny, despite the tennis. If you think about a seed, it is rather like a child. They both lie under the soil, seemingly dormant for a time, but secretly they are absorbing the world around them and metabolising it. They both are turning the outer muck into their inner foundations. And when they break out into sproutlings they are somehow more vulnerable for their success, to wind and ice and predators.

He is sitting at the table in the corner of the common room, bathed in the light that comes through the old Victorian windows that depress the energy efficiency rating of the school. He is like a houseplant with more complex emotions. He could be replaced with a fern (or a cactus, if it weren't for health and safety regulations). No one would be any the wiser.

And, like a houseplant, he exhibits extrasensory perception. Not always – it comes and goes, and maybe he wouldn't pass a scientific test, but there are some things beyond the grasp of science and always will be things a man in a white lab coat cannot validate.

When active, his ESP links him discreetly to the root cause of whatever he looks at. He can see, for example, the red thread running from his ankle to his mother and from his mother, under the sea, to yonder Nigeria, where it splits and dives into the ground at the sites where his predecessors are interred. It disturbs him to see their faces, to see how foreign he is to them. In evolution, children must look like their parents, but that is where the fealty ceases: go back a generation or three and they are alien.

There is a baseline unpleasantness with this experience, but

that is to be expected: things that are otherwordly are never rec-
onciled quite so neatly. There was the bad month, three months
ago, lost to guilt. Lost to weeping and mourning over all those
Black men, in America, dead, because of him. Every police officer
had said they'd seen his face and that's why they did it. It should
have been him. Each time. And the juries agreed. They'd all seen
his face and they saw a monster. A simple mistake to make, each
and every time. And he'd thought if only he could go there, and
get seen, and get shot, he would save all the others. And it crushed
him, it gnarled his insides to be stuck in school, in England, where
he couldn't get a gun for love or money.

* * *

The family is on holiday in Venice (or rather, they are accompany-
ing his father to a conference). With his mother, he has wandered
the streets of the sinking city. His father is busy with conference
work all day, work they wouldn't be interested in or understand,
so they have to kill the hours left empty without him. His mother
knows Venice, and to his surprise, in fact, speaks fluent Italian, but
will not be drawn into a conversation why. He finds he knows very
little about his parents' past. He heard once, at a family reunion,
that he has a vanished aunt. Years ago, as a teenager, his aunt supposedly travelled to Italy from Nigeria by herself and disappeared.
He doesn't see her absence in her mother or in any of his other
aunts or uncles. He finds himself suddenly taken by the fear that if
he were to disappear too they wouldn't give that away, either.

His mother is taking him to the golden house. His mother is
saying that his father will meet them at a party to celebrate the
conference later. His mother is showing him what it looks like as
he has never seen a picture of the art museum before. The golden
house faces out into the water, resplendent. Downstream, next
year, a refugee will drown with people pointing and laughing.

She explains to him that the golden house is really an old palace, that changed hands over and over again over the years. Each owner destroyed a small part of it before it was given away to the Italian state. She tells him she prefers the Basilica down the road, would rather be in the house of God, but is able to bear the smaller, humbler palace. She tells him they're only there to get away from the crowds, that she can't stand crowds, but really she means she can't stand the men, who leer and make comments she won't translate. It defies belief that they'd do that in a sacred place. It's irreverent.

She takes them to the foyer and encourages him to have a look around by himself. They separate, and he wanders alone. He crosses the square inner courtyard, with its grey stone fountain and its history set into the unassuming bricks there. He notes the braided vines that drape over the walls in exactly the same way a reclining panther crosses its paws. They are thick and grape-leaf green and give the impression that they own the place.

He comes to a small black statuette of Apollo and stares at it. He is trying to draw meaning from the golden hair and golden cloak and the blank stare. He feels like there should be something, that the composition will sing to him, reveal its secrets. But perhaps it has not deemed him worthy of conversation: he can only see silence. There is nothing there for him. Next year, during his Latin A-Level, they will miraculously come across Zeno, and he will see what he was missing.

Presently, he is joined in his efforts by another, whom he only acknowledges from the corner of his eye. A tourist is standing too close to him, his gaze fixed on *l'Antico*. This man is tall and thin, dressed in airy linens and flip-flops and dark curls all over him. His backpack is overloaded and the compact plastic camera around his neck is papered with stickers or stamps or something he can't quite make out unless he turns and looks properly.

Something is telling him it would be awful if he did, if he turned just a fraction. It is bizarre to him, but he instinctively knows it is forbidden, and there would be consequences, and it would not look good for anyone involved.

Suddenly, he feels claustrophobic – there is something else there, with the man, and the Apollo. It is around his chest and it's shrinking, and he can't breathe, and tears are welling up in his eyes. He leaves the man behind and walks very swiftly to the toilet, where he is sick. He has only vomited a little bit, little pale orange lumps, which flushed without complaint. He has only just wiped the remains from the corners of his mouth with toilet paper when the man from before enters the bathroom. And this time he sees him and he understands what is happening. He drops the crumpled tissue into a bin and then the tourist is upon him. The camera's hard corners dig into his chest and it hurts and he grimaces. The tourist whispers a quick sorry in French and relents. The taste of him in his mouth recedes for a moment. He is pulled into a stall – they are all empty. They expose themselves to one another. He is a mess of sensations and then it is over, then he needs to wash his hands again (and luckily, only his hands). The man smiles, says *au revoir*, leaves. It dawns on him that something significant has happened. He is left there to clean up.

As he is washing his hands, he notices a knife by the basin. It is khaki-green, handle to tip. It is like the knife that Will showed him once, on a Biology field trip, under the leafy cover of Epping Forest. It is the kind you'd buy if you actively prepared for the end of the world. Alarmed, he feels his chest – perhaps it wasn't the camera that dug between his ribs. But relief is at his fingertips: there is no wound. His shirt is now splattered dark from his wet fingertips. He scrunches paper towels into it hurriedly. If his mother saw the mess she would gently mock him, and he wouldn't quite be able to handle the normalcy of it, and he would cry. The water is dried and his shirt is crumpled, but he is satisfied. (He thinks he can tolerate her kissing her teeth at him.) He glances at the sink again. There is no knife.

He meets his mother, who has found the Apollo. Still, he sees nothing. They go back to the hotel.

Italian pop music drifts over the conference hall. It is like smoke that's been blown in from outside and is now settling. He doesn't know what the party is for. He is only there to show that his father has a family, a nice one worth looking at and enquiring about. *Who is he now?* And he has rehearsed the answer. He wants to be just like his dad. He loves the city. He is working hard.

This satisfies them. He is left alone, otherwise.

And then at that party something inside him switches on and he has to be somewhere else, away from everyone there and away from all that music. He has to be separate and distinct and outside and foreign. It itches, like a pox on the skin, to be a part of that gathering, to pretend he has something to say to anyone else there, or anything in common, that he can abide this ritual. And once removed, drunk and alone in the balmy night, he sees clearly that he's consigned to this. This is his lot. His fate is to wonder and mourn. He curses himself. He is such a wankstain. He can't go on like this, but cannot imagine another path. He is the lack of imagination, has no utopia within him, cannot envisage the milk or the honey. He remembers that they dug up a time capsule from the Soviet communists, and they thought they had won, that the common good would reign supreme and the Earth would be Eden again. And now it's him who's breaking their hearts; it's him who fails the covenant.

* * *

At home he is staring blankly at his Biology homework. He is in his room with the door closed. His room is four bare white walls, the decoration of his junior years scrapped and binned. Above the bed where he is sat now coalesce the sticky-taped, ripped fragments of poster paper and darker Blu-Tack marks, like the shadow of an old constellation. They are a sparse, spiralled trail of burned-out stars. His computer is on his lap and it is irradiating him. Radiation passes through you invisibly and changes you irreversibly. Radiation, for some futile millennia, keeps stars from imploding, before they become deep black holes.

He has been tasked with researching a presentation on photosynthesis. He has been paired with Julia. He doesn't want to just be in the way like all Julia's other partners have been. He wants to send her something she won't edit. He is to discover and then present how plants, through their leaves, sift through the boundless cosmic radiation which bathes all of us at all times. When they find light of the right wavelength, they turn it into food. They are gold-panners. They sway in a river imperceptible to the naked eye.

His room is rammed with novels, which have not been read for months. They persist in the four corners, in growing stalagmites. Before, he read fiercely. He theorised that if he consumed enough fiction, absorbed enough stories, he would grow something rich and worthy inside him. Now when he opens the page, the letters are a smear of dull glyphs it exhausts him to decipher. And so, the Biology homework, and the blank stare.

He shuts the laptop. He will not get anything done today. Frustration breaks out on his skin, an ugly, red rash on his chest. It reminds him he is powerless. He can only watch as this reality unfurls, indifferent to him.

He gets under the covers without turning off the lights. And then he sees large, tropical green fronds shiver out from the walls. His bed becomes a green mound, and his room a green expanse. He rises from the grassy knoll, beckoned by something unknown, and begins to walk. A peace, or perhaps an apathy, has fallen over him. He walks beyond the old confines of his room and his socks dissolve off his feet stitch by stitch, unwind and shuttle away, each thread worming into the warm earth which he feels singing beneath his toes. The green is now a mix of limes, pears, mosses, pickles, and emeralds. It swaddles him and wraps him in its gentle summer's aroma, making his mouth water.

The verdant space is perfumed with apricots, which punctuate the dizzying deep green with their colour. They have a rare sort of luminescence too, for they are streaking and spilling their ochre as light, making his head swim. They hang without trees, they are suspended only by the density of the foliage. The light of the apricots, and the garden, and now, from within him too, dances over his eyes, and over the plants, and over his soul. He walks further and further into the Eden. It welcomes him.

Here, a clearing. There is but grass, and bush, and silence.

Now, he is not alone. The force calling him home grows more intense. And the leaves of the bush before him shake, like an ecstatic drumroll, cheering *See! See! See!* And borne from the movement, from the anticipation, he sees Will, and Julia, and himself. And he sees that they love him, that other him, sweetly. The joy of it is like fruit, glowing with the goodness within. And they embrace each other, and apricots are growing in their hair, which is wild. And apricot means sunshine, really means sunshine, and you can see that in their cheeks and in their eyes. Those three give each other all the looks in the world. And they are looks full of poetry and lyric. And there, between them, there is a future.

Polychrome

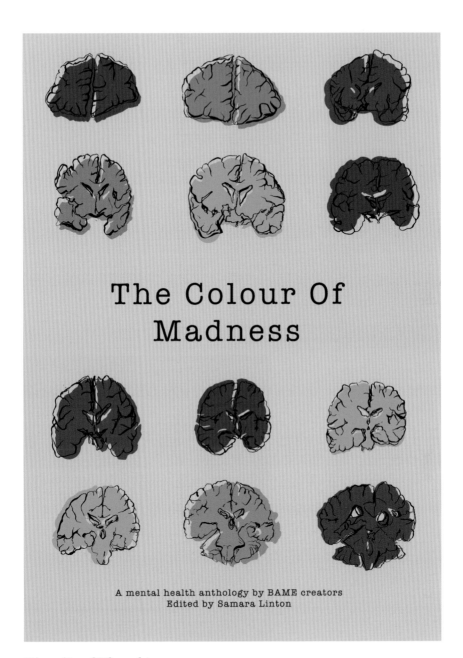

The Colour Of Madness

A mental health anthology by BAME creators
Edited by Samara Linton

Diversity of Thought
Neneh Patel

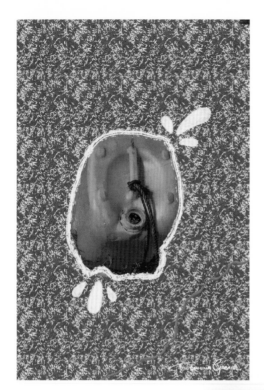

Spill
Theophina Gabriel
See Artist's Note, page 163

Ave Maria
Gold Maria Akanbi

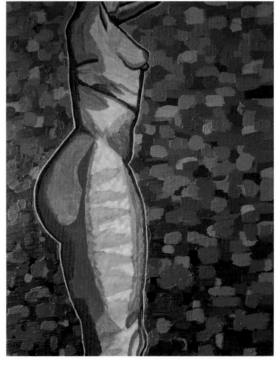

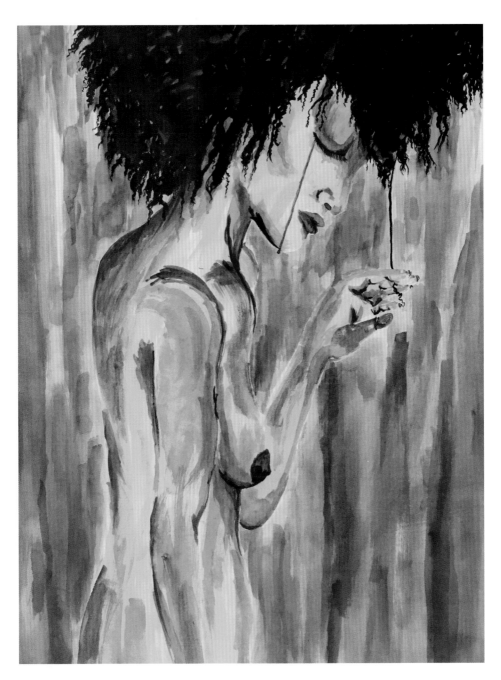

I Finger a Coil of my Hair and Tug

Farrah Riley Gray

See Artist's Note, page 164

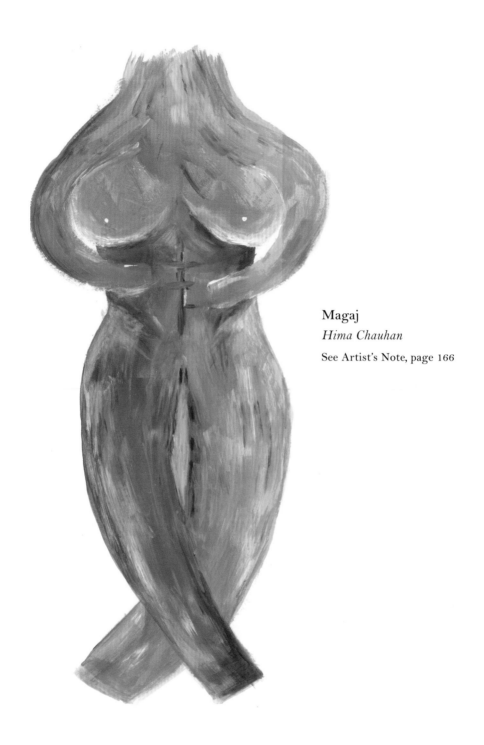

Magaj
Hima Chauhan
See Artist's Note, page 166

Utter it
Tobi Nicole Adebajo

Utter it.
Speak your truth into existence
Affirm your beautiful, brown resistance

Utter it.
Let the words flow uncensored
Reclaim the grounds upon which
your mothers' backs were bled senseless

Utter it.
Because your voices create waves -
templates for living, loving, being

Utter it.
Pick at the stitches
That have held your tongues,
and kept your lips from flowering
those seamless dances that you so often dream

Utter it.
Give your heart the space it needs
to move you along with its steady beat

Ultimately, silence. will. not. save. you.

Boohoo, poor you.
And your tantrum,
surprise...
At the fact that I was ready,
protected
And seated at the table
Ready when you decided
to catch up to your emotions,
To acknowledge the tumultuous nature
of your being,
To open your eyes to how you
swept me in your waves,
Watching my body fling between jagged rocks,
through untameable storms
Without so much as a thought for my being
No care for just how long it takes
for bones to reset

But by the time the winds had calmed,
life lulled back to rest

I was prepared,
Protected,
Ready,
Seated at the table

A Seat at the Table
Tobi Nicole Adebajo

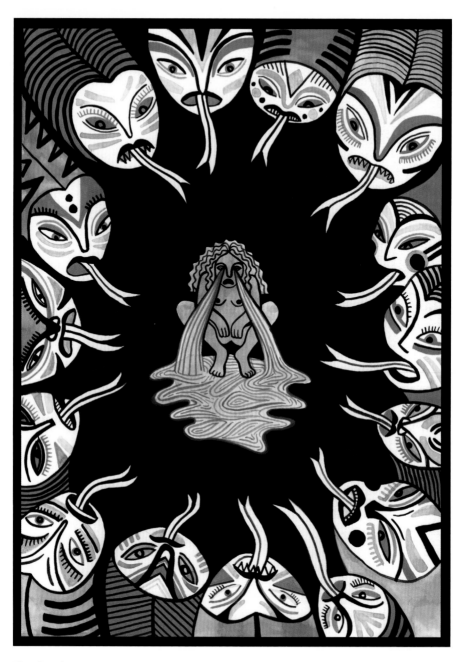

I'm Awake

Sophie Bass

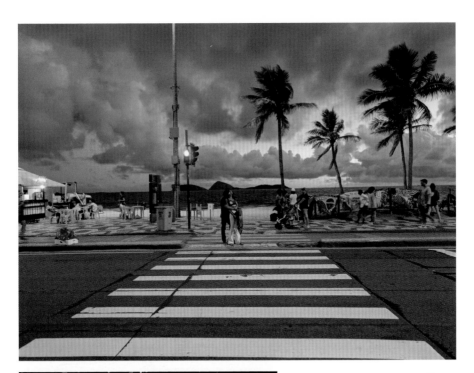

Love
Cynthia Oji

Mended Heart
Reba Khatun

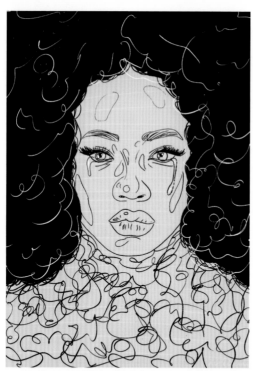

The History of Yellow
Avila Diana Chidume

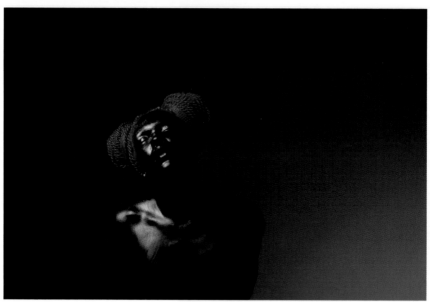

Untitled, The Beautiful Black Series, 2020
Gold Maria Akanbi

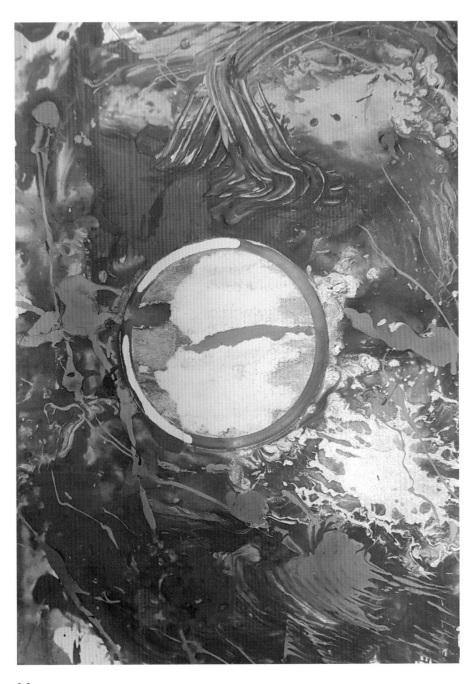

Moon

David Sohanpal

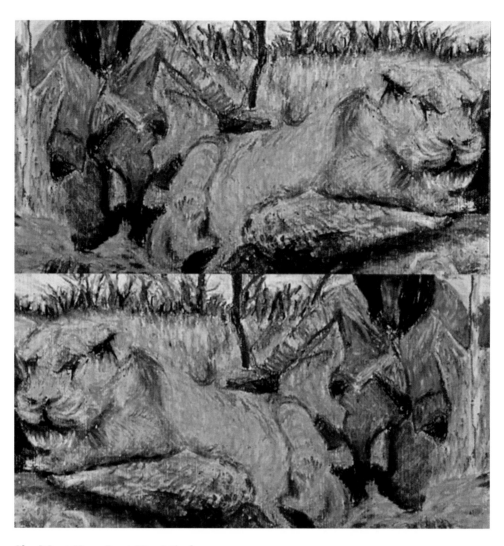

She Must Have Lost Her Mind

Corinne Crosbourne, aka 'thewomanistwords'

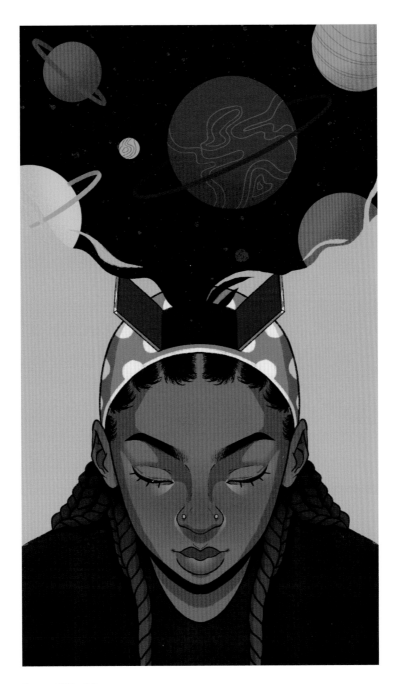

Inner World

Tosin Akinkunmi

See Artist's Note, page 168

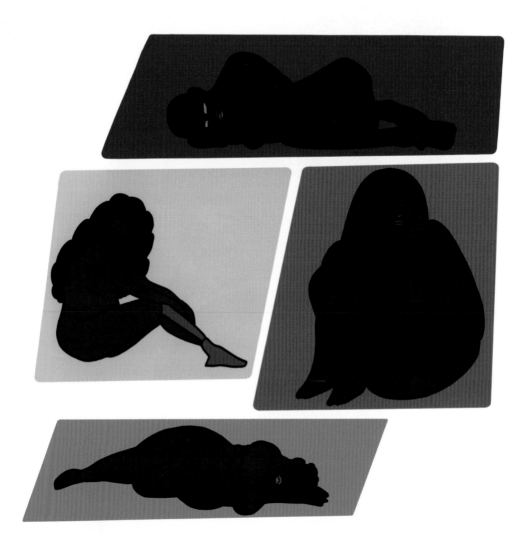

Ableism is

Tobi Nicole Adebajo

See Artist's Note, page 169

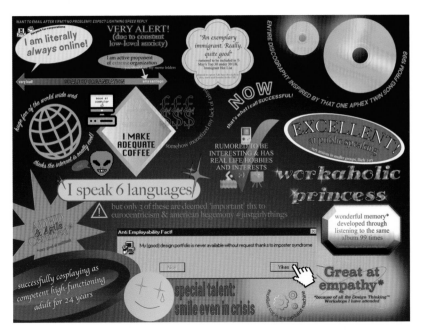

Personal Statement

Aimen Rafique-Marsh

See Artist's Note, page 171

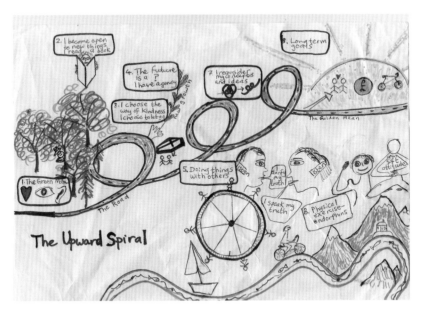

The Upward Spiral

Raza Griffiths

See Artist's Note, page 172

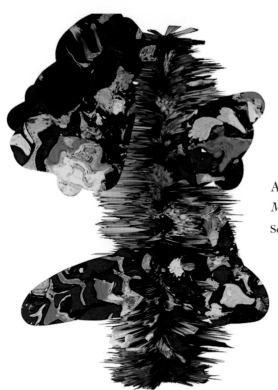

Animal Print
Michele D'Acosta
See Artist's Note, page 177

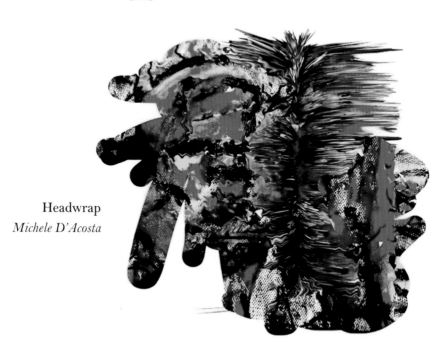

Headwrap
Michele D'Acosta

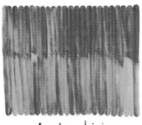

catastrophising

minimisation

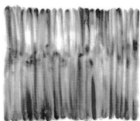

Personalisation

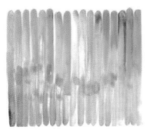

emotional reasoning

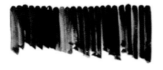
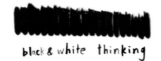

black & white thinking

overgeneralisation

Cognitive Distortions in Colour

Miz Penner-Hashimoto

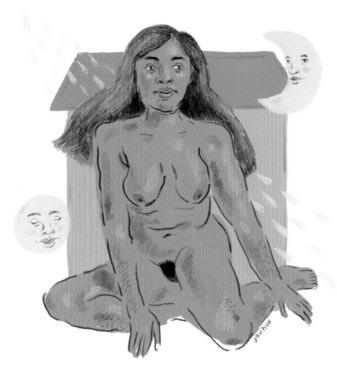

Seasons
Javie Huxley
See Artist's Note, page 179

We Rise
Maïa Walcott
See Artist's Note, page 180

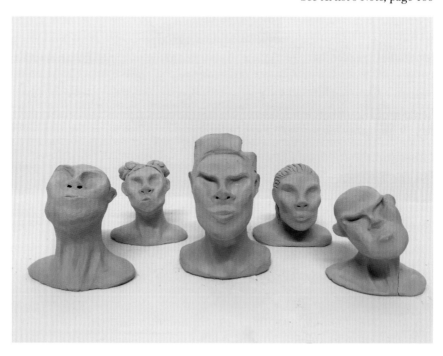

Artists' Notes

Some artists have written statements to accompany their work.

Spill

Theophina Gabriel

'Spill' taps into the concept of the body, and especially the mind, as water. It is a subtle look at the machinations of capitalistic structures that trap and affect our mental health. What does it mean for our minds to be contained within these structures and commodified as a resource? The small Black face drowns in itself, but simultaneously shows an opening; in us lies the chance for liberation, not found in the reformed action of being poured, but in the radical toppling of spilling free.

I Finger a Coil of my Hair and Tug

Farrah Riley Gray

My Black skin is not the picture of depression.
We are expected to be strong,
To suffer in silence.
So scared of being diagnosed,
Told to pray,
Do Russian Ballet,
Eat Blueberries.

Have you ever sat in a hospital waiting room,
After trying to kill yourself,
And been made to feel like a criminal?
I see how they treat that pretty White girl and me
    differently.

I'm ushered out of A & E,
Without being seen by a doctor,
Still bleeding.
I smear my heritage on the walls,
Castrated by the stereotype of Angry Black Woman.

My social worker calls,
He says 'Negro' on the phone to me.

My sick note has my ethnic background as 'White',
Can they not see the colour of my skin?
They tell me it doesn't matter,
They told me I don't matter,
Even though trauma is woven into the fabric of my skin.
If I pull the loose threads will I come undone?
I finger a coil of my hair and tug.

Magaj

Hima Chauhan

This painting illustrates the mutation of a woman of colour after an experience of rape. Through this medium, I depict how I viewed my body following this trauma. Consequently, I explore the relationship between a raped body and a survivor's mind. The cultural stereotype of South Asian women as dependent, and the incessant objectification and exotification of their bodies, greatly contributed to this expression. There is a sense that the body is guarding itself, while simultaneously conveying a sense of vulnerability and powerlessness. Under threat, the ambiguity in melanin signifies a confused and intemperate state of mind. In this piece, I invite you to consider how trauma can transcend mind and body, and the disturbance it creates in one's soul.

Postscript

Observing this painting now, I feel nothing. At first, I assumed years of therapy and time with myself meant that I had processed and overcome my trauma. Surely this is the grassier, greener side? Little did I know how destructive disassociation could be. While I was painting, I had a relatively open conversation with the disturbance inside me. However, now with a disassociated mind, it is like conversing with a ghost who doesn't care. Disconnection of mind and body can manifest in many ways, like retelling trauma to therapists as stories. I feel empathy for the main character, but they feel so far away. I look at this painting now, and I see another person.

Upon reflection, I understand that disassociation is an inbuilt function of survival. This breakdown in memory means I am not reliving my horrors every day. But by disassociating from real life, I became vulnerable and suffered a huge breakdown in my identity. Initially, I used materialism to create an illusion of belonging and entitlement. I called the aesthetic 'rich white woman'. Capitalising on the South Asian community's toxic love for status and success, I constructed my put-together identity. Funnily, this worked for a while, but my identity and bank were in crisis.

When the external and internal feel so far away, it is astonishing how you can lose yourself. Disconnecting left me vulnerable to the needs and wants of others, and so I had to find myself again. It is solely friendships with women that helped me heal. I feel at home when I am with my sister, my mom, Afrin, Ceridwen, and Alysha, to name a few. They tended to me, loved me unconditionally and saw me as a whole. They said, 'Hima, you are trying to figure yourself out, and I am here on that journey with you. I know you, and you are not so far gone. You are not trying to reach some abstract headspace where your mind and body connects and your sense of self aligns. You are just trying to come back to yourself, which is easier because you are here. I love you always.'

We are never that far from home.

Inner World

Tosin Akinkunmi

This piece is the best way I can articulate my creativity. As an autistic person, I sometimes find it difficult to fully articulate how and why I create what I create. It's easier to illustrate how that feels. Outwardly, I may not be particularly expressive, but inwardly, I feel like my imagination, and the creativity that stems from it, is boundless.

Ableism is

Tobi Nicole Adebajo

Ableism.
Ableism is,
Ableism is killing us
Ableism is killing me . . .

. . . it makes me forget when parts of my body are Off-limits and
Swollen.
Distended and Aching from the Pain that my joints are
experiencing.

I forget that my wrist has been subluxed for seven hours.
So, I Reach down to pull open that drawer where I keep my
batteries
See, the scale needs new batteries because my child wants us to
make pancakes

But those intrusive thoughts say:
'you absolutely cannot, MUST NOT! bake without a scale' . . .

. . . yes, yes, I understand that making pancakes is not exactly
'baking'

But there's 'cake' in the name
So, thank you, OCD brain . . .

. . . anyhow, I digress

Ableism is killing us,
Ableism is killing me,
Ableism kills,
Ableism is . . .
. . . and now, I've dislocated my wrist, again.

Personal Statement

Aimen Rafique-Marsh

Since coronavirus took my full-time corporate hustle, I've been OUT THERE, HuStLiNg, SELLING M?YSELF 24x7. Always with one-page resumés and cover letters and personal statements. But I am a Thinker, so it got me Thinking. When condensing myself to a page of 'experience' and 'accomplishments', what facets of ability are actually being celebrated? What constitutes the 'Personal' in my Personal Statements?

Thinking about it, much of the manifestations of my anxiety or ADHD help me assimilate and pass as a *Bonafide High-Functioning Competency Level 5000 Adult*™. But is this ability or just symptoms of chronic anxiety? Should I be celebrating various points of economic access that neurodiversity can grant me? Should I be asking for more in a typical workplace? Should we all be comfortable monetising all our accidental skills and used-to-be-hobbies? (Are they still hobbies?) Maybe it's just been a while since I used Times New Roman in a project, and that's all this is about.

'Personal Statement' is a digital collage and anti-capitalist narrative questioning the glamorisation of workaholicism and 'being busy'.

The Upward Spiral

Raza Griffiths

1. The Green Man

In the aftermath of a life crisis, my feet draw me to the Green Wood. Here, I sense the presence of a mystical woodland figure, called The Green Man. He is the dweller in the deep of the Green Wood.

When I am extremely quiet and still, I feel him as a gentle breeze on my face, I hear him in the leaves rustling in the wind, and I feel him as an elusive presence in my heart.

I cannot summon his presence at will and he appears only when he wants.

2. I become open to new things

But when I do feel his presence, I feel expanded and spacious. I am more open to experiencing new things, and can even take pleasure in reading a book. The next book I will read is by Neil MacGregor, *Germany: Memories of a Nation*. It looks at the history of Germany through a series of physical objects.

3. I choose the way of kindness. I choose to let go.

These affirmations become real when I am in the Green Wood. Here, I am able to meet my grief and acknowledge my pain and loss – whether it is the ending of a relationship or the destruction of childhood – and put it in a different place in my life. This is symbolised by the coffin.

At this point, a branch of wood grows out of my hand and sprouts delicate, silky, green leaves. And I feel how loss is just one part of the life cycle, and that I can be open to the possibility of new growth.

4. The future is an open book – I have agency

I begin to feel the future is an open book. I no longer feel I am helpless, but that I have a sense of agency, albeit in a world that is bigger than I am and ultimately out of my control.

5. Doing things with others

I no longer feel isolated and feel open to any number of possibilities for meaningful communion with others. I am, after all, a social being!

The circle symbolises my coming together with others as equals in meaningful and satisfying activity.

More specifically, it is a bicycle wheel representing my membership of a cycling group where I feel accepted and valued. We regularly cycle 50 miles, and it boosts my self-confidence to know I can do this. When cycling, I feed my senses with the beauty of the countryside. I am in good company, and the endorphin rush from physical activity gives me a natural high.

The wheel also symbolises a birthday cake I baked and shared with the wider collective of my extended family. They enjoyed my company and my cake, and they may well ask me to bake cakes for future birthdays. This feedback loop gives me a sense that I am valued, and not just for my cake!

On a broader level, the wheel symbolises my current work for a mental health peer-support and campaigning group for people from Black and Minority Ethnic communities. We meet around the circle and support each other as equals, and we connect with ever-widening constellations of people who share our passion for campaigning for social justice. In this example, the circle becomes the universe, or our wider social, economic, and political environment.

The river is the river of life, meandering through the countryside and culminating in some snow-capped mountains which house a retreat for spiritual development. There is a boat on the river, even though life is not always plain sailing!

6. Clarifying and speaking my truth

In the course of me being with others and engaging in meaningful activity with them, an internal process occurs, which started with the Green Man, and which leads to me being able to articulate with complete clarity, the complex emotions, thoughts, feelings, psychical imprints, and memories that had formerly overwhelmed me. It is as if a heavy weight, which had previously produced a sinking downwards vortex in my being, is transformed into a delicately petalled flower swaying in the breeze. And I am in communion with others who are able to hear me. And there are many more of them than I ever thought possible, some of them people near me whom I never felt able to talk to before. And I, in turn, am able to hear them articulate their truth.

7. *I reconsider my concepts and ideas*

While honouring my thoughts and feelings about my past, I am able to reconsider the ways I had previously labelled and understood myself. ('Where did these ideas come from?' is a question for another time.) I feel that I have the power to reshape and change them to meet my emerging sense of self.

I am no longer trapped and immobilised within a circular prison by the thunderbolts of the Lightning Hurlers (a process I describe in Raza's Mandala); nor am I any longer a marginalised victim at the painful intersection of overlapping circles (this process is described in the Circles of Victimhood). Instead, the circles of these former ways of understanding myself have unravelled like the skin of an unpeeled orange, which becomes the Upwards Spiral.

8. *Physical exercise*

I am still aware that, despite being on my journey, my mind continues to live in an internal and external environment that is toxic. I focus more on my body, which I had previously neglected.

I feed it through strenuous exercise. In doing so, mind and body are brought into wholeness. I have to be careful though, of not overdoing it. I am mindful of making physical exercise into a mere tool, a means to an end through gritted teeth – albeit for the positive end of wellness. I consciously sink myself into enjoyment of the exercise, in the moment of doing it.

9. *Future goals*

In the course of my journey along the Upwards Spiral, I feel a sense of uplift. But I am aware that my journey cannot always be going upwards and that life will continue to have its ups and downs. At some point, the road will level out to meet the line of the horizon. This is the golden mean.

But on that horizon, borne of spaciousness, there now appear a series of visions that I can work towards. There is a vision of two men holding hands, a golden coin, and a bicycle. These signify respectively, the possibility of being in a relationship – or more broadly, of being in harmonious relationship with myself, other people and the universe; of being wealthy – or having a sense of plenitude in my life and not being in hardship or want; and of continuing to cycle, despite my physical impairments which are hindering my cycling – or, more broadly, of having the continued ability to move forward on my journey of life and discovery.

The fact that I am able to conjure up these visions and believe in them is an affirmation of the fact that I am no mere animal, living a hand-to-mouth existence, surviving emotionally from moment to moment. In the course of my journey along the Spiral, I have experienced a new and life-affirming truth about myself.

Animal Print and Headwrap

Michele D'Acosta

In my early twenties, when I began to express my personal experiences through multimedia, I found myself in an autobiographical dilemma. I had yet to become socially and politically conscious of the African and Black diaspora that informed my artistic roots. As a result, I faltered when I realised that the Eurocentric linear narrative formula could never adequately explain what I was feeling. So, I searched for an art form to combine the diaphanous threads of my lost African Mother Tongue, my Eurocentric scholastic disciplines, and my vivid childhood growing up in the post-punk musical era – a child under the influence of The Clash and The Sex Pistols and the clash of cultures.

My early training as a dancer gave me the courage to investigate and discover that it is vital to find a common universality, a non-linear language. The following years were immersed in transcribing what I felt to be messages from a distant past: layers of identity crossing boundaries and stirring my cellular memory. It took several years before my instincts led me to experiment with visual storytelling and the superimposition of images – a discovery which freed me from the constraints of linear structure.

By employing superimposition and interweaving layers of sound, photography, painting, storytelling and moving images, I found a way to excavate my ancestral memory and translate this into a hybrid creative identity.

The versatile nature of superimposition allows me to collage, sample and reinterpret my connection to past and present. When I reimagine traumatic experiences in a positively charged context, I endeavour to recalibrate old energies; to create a space for us all to reappraise and re-evaluate what has been lost over time.

Seasons

Javie Huxley

I created this illustration in the first lockdown in the UK. The illustration is a response to feeling trapped in many senses by the pandemic and pre-existing anxieties that were heightened by the months inside. Despite this, I felt moments of respite when I looked out of my window and saw the changing of seasons. We slowed down, but nature continued its comforting cycles.

We Rise

Maïa Walcott

Since moving to a new city and studying at a predominantly white university, I have – for a while now – felt hyper-visible, haunted by the feeling of being observed. Occasionally, I even manage to convince myself that the moment I turn my back, heads collectively swivel in my direction, fixating their glossy eyes on the nape of my neck, which grows hot with anxiety and embarrassment.

Enrolling in a sculpture course where I was the only Black person only amplified this feeling. The space of my art class reflected that of the art world – marked by its lack of diversity. In reaction to this, I encouraged myself to confront and reshape ideas about which bodies belong at the centre of the art world. In my sculpture work, I attempted to subvert Eurocentric, normative standards of beauty and body shape by crafting bodies and forms that are marginalised. In this art class, I began to sculpt a series of maquettes in resistance to the whiteness of the space around me.

I hand-carved these maquettes from clay and designed them to have distinctly Black features: sharp cheekbones, strong brow lines, shaped hairlines and wide nose bridges. I decided to accentuate these features in the hopes of challenging and disrupting norms of European beauty in art, and particularly sculptures and busts. I also created these sculptures to normalise the artistic rendering of Blackness and to place them firmly at the centre of sculpture practice. When sculpting, I am purposeful with each stroke and nudge of my thumb as I create reflections of my own body and the bodies that surround me, making more inclusive and truthful art. Through creative expression, my art allows me to challenge my learned preconceptions of the body. Seeing reflections of myself in the art that I create is validating and empowering because it allows me to assert my presence in the artistic spheres I am part of.

In other corners of the classroom, different representations of Blackness were taking form. One student recreated a collection of golliwog dolls she had found in her grandfather's house from twisted wire and string, bringing to life her vision of the Black body. At the front of the classroom, the teacher used me as his muse, carving my likeness into a wooden sculpture that would end up in an art show on the European continent, with no credit to the anonymous Black woman that inspired the piece. Amid this art school in Edinburgh, an imperial centre in denial of its roots, a new triangle was forming. One student crafting hyperbolic caricatures of Blackness, the teacher sculpting me, and I, sculpting Black busts rising above transatlantic waters. In the midst of hypervisibility and surveillance, and the repeated artistic objectification of Black 'self' into 'Black body', I challenged the loss of personhood implicit in white observation of Blackness by infusing my art with vitality.

While creating my maquettes, I exaggerated traditionally Black features without reducing them to caricatures, while the white student simply recreated and reproduced symbols from my oppressive history. As the only Black student in the space, I hoped that someone, perhaps the teacher, would intervene and protect me. Instead, the other students placidly clapped and praised her ingenuity. As the teacher complimented the work with no further comments, I felt isolated, panicking, bewildered at this culture of silence in which the whole classroom became complicit.

I chose to break the silence.

'Those dolls on top of your grandad's cabinet should have remained there.'

The wide white eyes of the golliwog dolls followed me as I left the room, raising the hairs on the back of my neck.

Blue

Sometimes, we see in blue. We see through sharp
frames, smart collars, and the towering walls of
institutions.

Things My Therapist Does Not Know

Haania Amir Waheed

My therapist tells me
That to get through a panic attack
I must reach for a glass of water,
And allow myself to shake and shudder
Let the water spill
Over the lip of the glass
And seep past mine
Into the back of my throat where I allow it to choke me.
I must remember that panic attacks are normal
And remind myself I am not in any danger,
Because the reminder should stop me from sinking
Into the abyss of my frantic fears.

What my therapist doesn't know
Is that I drowned six months ago.

My therapist tells me
That I need to *trust* my friends, my family
That when I allow myself to fall,
It should be into the arms of their expectations
Which I have always been too short for.
When I come up inadequate, with

The nails of their disgust scraping at my pride,
Rings of blood still contouring my eyes
She tells me I need to trust my *friends*, my *family*.

What my therapist doesn't know
Is that in the fall
Trust burst into a thousand fragments.
Its bones need electroshock therapy,
There's little chance of recovery.

My therapist tells me
That sometimes, when people face a great tragedy,
When their insides are blackened,
Their hearts grated and stringy,
It's normal for them to be alone but not feel lonely.
She tells me that tragedies come in many
Different forms, and mine might not feel grand
But I should remember that it broke me,
And the times when all my ribs held was a bowl of grief
    and melancholy,
It was not my imagination, but depression and anxiety.

But she doesn't know
That my head was stuffy and muted because
Pulling away from everyone called 'friend'
Had turned into an obsessive duty,
And the seldom nights when I had an appetite
I was eating the darkness,
Hoping to catch a taste of light.

My therapist tells me
That as an attractive young lady

I should not shy away from the attention
The curves of my lips get me.
The blush on my cheek shouldn't be eclipsed
By the red of my mortification,
And the throb in my chest
Should not be fear
But flattery
When I am told I am beautiful
By a stranger in the street.
After all, she says, he complimented me.

What she doesn't know is
I am allergic to the word 'beautiful'.
That I have been trying to be more than my face.
Taller than my small-scaled facade,
And between my legs there's this space
That has made me smaller
Than my 4 feet 11 inches.

My therapist tells me
That I am strong and selfless.
In my weakest moments of insecurity
When every social media story
Pricks at my veins,
Makes my fingers itch for a razor blade
She says I need to be compassionate
To myself.

What she doesn't know is
I don't need a fresh blade
To cut at my face, because

The scars from my last admirer
Spell out 'tease' on my face.

My therapist tells me
That someday I will feel
Again
The pain I should've known
When my breastbone kept on bruising.
I expected my collarbone would burst
As did the cysts in my ovary.
The doctor said I was numb,
It hid from me my misery.
This nothingness I feel
Is my body taking a break from the stress.
Maybe it is fighting hard for sanity,
When every recklessly drawn breath in my lungs
Itches to rattle and wheeze around my body.
Shuddering with my fingertips
As I crawl to a corner heaving,
The haze of steam that envelops every one of my feelings
The one that blurs the sadness with the healing
Detaches me from the smile on my lips
And the endless stream of nonsense text messages.
And so my therapist tells me
My subconscious is protecting me.

What she doesn't know is
I am not worth defending.

When my therapist told me
Being home would make me feel again,
I stopped sitting in that armchair

across from her and pretending
I didn't want to adopt
all
non-verbal cues of
being closed-off and
use Freud and Skinner
on her
instead of nodding along.

Because when she said
That it was homesickness
Which explained my physiological pain,
The breaks in my breaths
The flagged in red blood tests and
The days I would be shackled to my bed
I knew I couldn't tell her
What she doesn't know
My greatest secret of all –
There's nowhere I belong.

Postscript

'Things My Therapist Does Not Know' was written after a very difficult period of my life. It wasn't written during, when all writing and self-expression escaped me, and it wasn't written with a realisation that things had been tough. I had simply put words on paper to express myself.

I only realised the gravity of what I had been through when I read the poem out to my then-flatmate, D. Sitting on her bedroom floor, a foot away from me, my ever-energetic and radiant friend burst into tears. D said she was crying because she knew I had been through a lot in that past year but hearing me *describe* what it felt like *inside* was what got her.

It hadn't gotten to me. If anything, I didn't feel much when performing these words in front of hundreds of people at poetry slams. Things changed a year later when I was back home, in a safer place, and I read this at a poetry slam. The audience's response was incredible. Yet, I felt dirty. It felt wrong to use these feelings in a poem at a slam and unjust that I had had to write them at all.

This poem was later adapted for *The Colour of Madness: A Play*[13] and was included in the NEON Collection, an NHS study researching the benefits of mental health narratives in recovery processes.[14] I remember feeling incredibly hesitant; why would someone find peace and healing in an admission of such statelessness?

Years down the line, when Rianna and Samara wrote to us about this second edition, I saw this as my chance to say, 'Look, I made it!' That I could make it at all. And in lots of ways, I have. I made it to my career goals, goals that were years in the making; I feel confident to be my own practising Muslim minority self, wearing my shalwar kameez under the seldom-seen English sun, reconnecting with my language and culture with confidence. And yet, for me to write *that* afterword, from the voice of the Haania who made it, would be a lie. I wanted to use this edition to edit my poem with an unbiased, unaffected eye; but the truth is I haven't been able to reread it.

In many ways, I am back to that very difficult period that prompted this poem. However, there is a difference this time, and I hold it close to my chest. This time, I know *where* I belong.

On Becoming a Psychologist

Dr Cassie Addai

Growing up as a Black girl in a majority-white city, I can vividly recall examples of overt racism, including being teased because of my 'thick lips' and being told to 'go back' to where I 'came from'. Then, there were subtle, but equally painful incidents like being the only Black student in class when the word 'slavery' was uttered and feeling thirty pairs of eyes fixate upon me. I now know that systemic racism infiltrates our society so that experiences of marginalisation become an expected, and seemingly accepted, reality for Black people. As a child, I did not have the words to describe the cumulative effects of such interactions, but I had the emotions. Hurt, anger, and loneliness. I remember finding solace in books where I could learn about other people's stories and being amazed by people like Martin Luther King Jr and Rosa Parks. Their stories of strength in overcoming injustice captivated me.

The idea of strength is one that I have held on to for many years, but the concept of vulnerability appeared much later. Adolescence is, of course, a period of transition known for its challenges. It was during this time, against a background of exam stress, changing hormones, and identity struggles, that I suddenly became aware of my own vulnerability. I felt myself breaking down as I began to regularly experience shortness of breath, palpitations, sheer panic, and a feeling of disconnect from my surroundings. Having always felt in control of my body, I found myself suddenly doubting all that I had accepted as certain and questioning what was wrong with me. My mind jumped to physical explanations for these symptoms. Shortly after, the term 'mental health' was introduced to me during A-Level Psychology, and I became fascinated. Prior to this, I certainly had not considered mental health something that everyone has, in the same way that we all have physical health. As I learned about anxiety, I recall a huge sense of relief at finding an explanation for my experiences and learning just how common these difficulties are.

I was drawn to a career in psychology by a desire to be with people who are experiencing distress, hear their stories, and support them towards ways of coping. Ten years have passed, but I still hold those A-Level lessons in mind and recall how important they were in developing my understanding of mental health. Now, as a psychologist, I see the impact of our circumstances on our mental health and wellbeing. A wealth of research suggests that experiences of deprivation, abuse, unemployment, homelessness, isolation, discrimination, and other forms of adversity can negatively impact mental health. In sessions with clients, it is often these social explanations that people articulate when explaining what has brought them to psychological services. However, Psychology has historically held a more individualistic perspective of distress, which primarily focuses on increasing individuals' resilience to adverse situations through changing the way that they think and behave. I am increasingly aware of the disparity between what we know about the social causes of poor mental health and the individualised interventions we offer to those in distress. I am aware of how often this knowledge of social causes evaporates, leaving individual blame in its place.

I have heard colleagues dismiss and deny Black clients'

experiences of discrimination, unaware that, in doing so, they are perpetuating the very same acts of oppression that the client described. There are occasions when Black clients raise topics, such as the impact of being dark-skinned in a society that favours whiteness, and this is often left unacknowledged by the therapist. Alternatively, these clients are labelled as 'paranoid', which can contribute to the disproportionately high rates of psychosis diagnoses in Black clients. Rather than understanding the client's concerns as valid in the context of a society where institutional racism is rife, the Black client is positioned as 'crazy' or 'imagining things'. As such, what might be understood by the Black client as a normal response to the systematic discrimination they face, is pathologised by professionals as symptomatic of a mental health problem. The implicit message is that therapy is not a space to talk about race. Hearing and witnessing these examples takes me back to those early experiences of being Black in a majority-white context. The name-calling may have ceased, but there is still the challenge of negotiating racism in its many guises, and this time as an adult in a professional setting. Similar feelings of hurt, anger, and loneliness arise, but this time, those feelings fuel me to speak up.

I believe that Psychology must acknowledge its own role in racism, in particular, its foundations upon a white, Western, and individualistic knowledge base, which does not reflect the rich diversity of society. As a profession, Psychology seems to recognise that Black people are less likely to access mental health support than their white peers and, in response, there are initiatives to 'increase access' in the hope of redressing this inequality. However, I feel uncomfortable with the prospect of merely increasing the number of Black clients without true reflection on the ways in which systemic racism operates within Psychology itself.

I only have to look around at my colleagues to know that we do not represent the diversity of the UK nor the clients that we see. The majority of my peers are white and from middle-class backgrounds, and I know first-hand the struggle of broaching the topic of race with them, no matter how well-meaning they may be. Put simply, Psychology does not seem able to reflect on its race problem, and there seems to be little recognition of the challenges that this may present for people of colour whose daily experiences of being silenced risk continuation within the therapy room.

Although I was drawn to Psychology because of my interest in hearing people's stories, I am increasingly aware of the need for activism within my role. While listening to, and truly hearing, people's experiences is essential, I now realise that this, in itself, is not sufficient. Psychologists must also actively speak up against the systematic injustices, which wear down the mental health of people of colour, especially those who also occupy marginalised gender, sexuality, and class identities. One small way of doing this might be to ask about people's experiences of race and racism directly, including whether this has affected their wellbeing. We must step out from the profession's supposedly neutral and 'colour blind' stance to actively combat oppression. We must use our strength and relative privilege as mental health professionals to advocate for people of colour.

The Good Indian Nurse

Dr Kamal Kainth

I was old enough to know better this time. I may only have been fourteen, but I was already questioning whether a psychiatric ward was really the best place to leave Mum. It had become a familiar pattern: her highs, psychosis, suicide attempts followed by long hospital stays that swallowed up my school holidays and distracted me from my homework during term. But had she ever come out of the hospital feeling better? I wasn't so sure. Quieter, yes, but *better*?

There is a lot I don't remember from this particular incident: why she was sectioned, how long she spent as an in-patient. But I do remember that it was dark – evening, perhaps – and I remember the ward because of the familiar same decor. I had been visiting this unit since I was at least five.

This memory is silent, apart from a sentence or two whispered to my sister, and the goodbye that Mum ignored. Also, it has a colour – it is beige and orange, the sepia you would use as a filter on your phone. But this was in the early nineties; the only phones we had then were attached to the wall. If I try hard enough, I can also recall us sitting as a family in a grey room, waiting for the nurses to sort out a bed and formally admit her. We all sat there in a row, saying nothing. Mum held her head in her hands. There were bouts of tears, probably from all of us at some point, but it's Mum's silent tears that I remember the most.

We lived in a multicultural borough in west London, the patients were mostly white, but there were a few Black patients too. I imagine that even the units in the whitest suburbs have Black patients. The nurses were always white. Even when I visited the unit as a smaller, naive infant, I had picked up that these white surroundings would be alien to her.

The faces on the ward had largely become familiar, although not friendly. On this occasion, a woman walked out of the nurses' station. I watched her, wondering what she was doing back there. She was Indian, wearing faded black jeans and a jumper and looked about forty. I saw that she had keys as she wandered past me into the common area, and I realised that she was a nurse. She was an Indian woman, and she was a nurse. I feel stupid about this now, but in some unknowable way, it was a defining moment for me. I saw her, and I thought, it's okay to leave Mum here. Mum's going to be all right.

The official visiting window had closed hours ago – we had been permitted to stay longer – and it was time to go. It felt better this time because now Mum had an ally. Right? We left Mum sitting in a stained pleather chair in the common room. The Indian nurse was in there too, standing by the radiator. She didn't look up or acknowledge us. I stood in the corridor for a few minutes and watched them. It was hard to leave, hard to leave Mum there. I wanted some reassurance, however slight, that we had made the right decision in bringing her here again. The nurse walked away taking my hope with her. Why had I believed that their brown skin was enough to connect them?

I'm on the other side now, working in mental health services as a psychotherapist. I have worked on wards and in the community, and I am sure I have been the source of that same disappointment for others. Others that I did not see. I work hard, from the heart and in an open way, but I have overlooked people, patients, families. It would have been unintentional, but it would be silly to pretend that it hasn't happened.

Looking back, that Indian nurse had looked sad: who knows what was going on for her? I had believed and hoped for a connection in a glance. I think I just expected her to care (more?), and when she didn't, it confused me, shattered my fantasy of the Indian community. I still wonder if she stayed working in mental health. I wonder if she is okay. And I wonder what my brown skin means to the service users and their families who are faced with me as a mental health professional.

Asian on a White Ward in a White Town

Dylan Thind

As told to a family member.

I don't feel I have much to say, so maybe you can just ask me questions.

I was sectioned because I made a serious attempt on my life. I took an overdose, but managed to stay alive and woke up in the hospital, and I was sectioned after that. I've been sectioned since then, fourteen months.

I'd had a very traumatic experience before this, and I'm not sure I've got over it. My post-traumatic stress disorder (PTSD) is getting better, in that I don't have flashbacks anymore, but I think with extreme trauma, especially prolonged extreme trauma, you will always carry it with you.

I'm an Asian man in my thirties on a psychiatric ward in an almost exclusively white town in the South West of England.

I do feel like an outsider in this town and on this ward. And I do feel like I'm treated differently because of my race.

For example, I love hip-hop and other similar music. But there was an incident where I recommended a song called 'Gihad' by a rapper called Raekwon to one of the other service users. The staff – incorrectly – said I had recommended a Jihadi video. They didn't believe me when I said it wasn't, and they didn't check.

As a result of this, I got put under a one-to-one observation, when they monitor you for twenty-four hours a day and [isolate] you in your own room. I was also referred to the Prevent Programme safeguarding investigation, which they later abandoned because there was no substance to their claims.

I think they referred me because of the colour of my skin; they thought I was a Jihadi. I think it was also because I was growing a beard at the time. The staff talk in handovers but get a lot of things wrong.

Would I say this was racism? It's difficult to know for sure, but I'd guess that it was. There are Black agency staff, but no Black or Asian permanent staff actually work on the ward; they're all white. The ones that complained about me – they were all white. Currently, I am the only non-white patient on the ward and the longest-standing BME person.

So, that incident was the most glaringly obvious example of where I had been treated differently because of my race, but you don't know if you're being treated differently in more subtle ways. Like, if a white person would get away with something that I'd be told off for; you don't know it, but you *feel* it. I think I feel it in general in the South West; that being on a psych ward in here I just feel the racism.

It is difficult to quantify, but racism is always bubbling just under the surface. Even if patients are nice to you, you know that if you annoyed them or something went badly, they would turn to racism. So, you always have to be really careful. Especially with the harder, tougher patients.

There once was a guy that told me a very offensive, racist joke, I think to get a reaction from me. And there was another patient who thought I was a terrorist; she constantly asked me if I'd been to Guantánamo Bay. It made me feel like an outsider – someone that is not British. I tried to tell the staff about this, the head nurse, and she just said that the patient's very unwell at the moment. I think I always feel like an outsider, especially when I'm in the South West and more so on the ward. I think it's because I'm Asian and I do visually appear different to the other people on the ward. But there are some lovely patients on the ward who do include me.

Also, I remember the time one of my relatives asked me to change into my jeans from my tracksuit bottoms before we went out because it was cold. The nurse said, 'I don't know what they do in *your* culture, but in *our* culture, you can dress the way you want to.' My relative was just trying to help, so I didn't get cold outside.

You're asking me if being Black or Asian predisposes people to more mental health problems. It's a good question. From what I know, Black people are disproportionately more likely to develop schizophrenia, and Asian people are more likely to develop depression. It is so complex to try to work out exactly why this is, but I think that being visibly different makes you quite self-conscious and quite introverted, and these traits I think can lead to depression.

And I think when you get a lot of racist abuse, you turn anger inwards when you can't really fight back, and lots of anger turned inwards can lead to depression as well.

I really think that someone from a BME background living in a white town is likely to develop some sort of mental health issue. With me, I was trying to fight against it, but it inevitably caught up with me. When I had my trauma a few years ago, everything came up to the surface.

I don't feel that the white psychiatrist I've had from the start understands me. Everything I say he will dismiss as delusion. And he's convinced that antipsychotics will change my thinking. But my thinking is based on truth and my experiences, and no kind of pill can change what happened to me. I suppose therapy would be more conducive than a tablet.

The psychiatrist has a very pharmaceutical idea of happiness. He believes that ramping up the chemicals will solve my problems. He's very much 'by the book', and the things that I try to tell him, like about kundalini* experiences and things of that nature, get instantly dismissed as a delusion.

There are experiences outside the medical model that are just as valid. Kundalini is a Hindu thing. I think that's another reason why a white psychiatrist will not understand the experiences of someone from a different culture. A more modern, open one could, but they would have to be someone who really does their research about all sorts of experiences.

There is a Black psychiatrist who is not that much better but seems more caring. But he also just sanctions more pills. I do think that some of this is the result of [being in a provincial town]. The majority of nurses have never lived away from here – it's true, I've asked – and so, they've never really had their experiences broadened by other cultures, by other art, by other knowledge.

I find boredom on the ward the most difficult thing to deal with. When the kundalini left my body, or when I developed psychosis, it took away all my creativity, so now I find it very difficult to write – which is why you are writing this up for me. And I find it hard to do all the things that used to keep me occupied. It made my mind quite slow and sluggish, so now I have a tendency to be bored a lot.

You're telling me that what I'm saying and have told you shows someone who is very creative and articulate. I don't feel it's creative.

---

* Kundalini, a Sanskrit word meaning coiled serpent. It refers to the primal, creative energy that is said to reside at the base of the spine.

I'd like to have more things to do on the ward. At the moment, we all just feel contained, we're given no real help. When you ask one of the staff for something, they act like they're doing you a favour. A lot of the time, they'll ask you to wait for five or ten minutes, and when you look inside the office, they're doing nothing but having a chat. There have been good nurses, but I find all the best ones tend to leave. There is one great activity coordinator because he really cares. More caring staff would be good.

The staff could be more empathic. There seems a lack of empathy on the ward. If someone is crying, most of the staff will just walk past them and not do anything. It last happened yesterday with a girl called Julie who is very emotional and cries a lot. I don't think she gets treated well by the staff; they don't know how to handle her.

For example, there was one time she was sick in the toilets and rather than asking her if she was okay, or if she needed anything, the nurse just said, 'Have you just been sick? You've missed a bit, clean it up,' and was really angry at her. The nurse shouted it in front of everyone in the corridor. Julie started crying. She gets bad anxiety, which was why she was sick. She's only very young.

Everyone is bored in here, and they don't know what to do with their time. I want to be discharged, but they have not given me a definitive date. They must think I'm a risk to myself, but I don't think I am now. I feel better. Although I don't feel as good as I used to feel.

I used to have a really good job before the trauma. Before, I was working for what was considered at the time the best start-up to work for. My mind was working very sharply; I was able to do very complex coding work. It wasn't mania; it was kundalini. I lived in a really cool part of the city, had great housemates and lots of friends.

Now things are completely different. Before, if I checked my

Facebook, there would be ten or eleven invites for all sorts of arty things. Now, I don't have invites for anything. If you're out of the city for long enough, you just get forgotten about. But I have a lot of friends who still contact me and stay true to me.

In the future, I'd like to be discharged and slowly be able to build my life again. My friends and family would help me build my life again; having something to work on, like a project, would help. I think the future's going to be hard: I've changed and will always carry the scars. But I hope things can get better.

Incognito

A. K. Niemogha

Day 2: the start of my journey to anew, I visited a strange place.
There was a man, with skin that resembled mine, but a mind
seen sadly as flawed.
I've been told to fear men like this; for their dark skin and dark
thoughts,
They are a danger to society – danger to myself.
My pulse quickened as we gazed at one another; did he know
my secret?

Day 19: I travelled with a friend to another strange place.
It was described as a place to heal; no harm could come to
persons there.
Again, I was met with the man I saw on day 2 of this journey.
This time his gaze burnt an opening to my mind,
I know he knows my secret now.

The man argued with all that sat around him, but I remained
silent.
Repeatedly he proclaimed that he would stand for himself,
Repeatedly he stated that no man had the best of intentions
for him.

No freedom to leave the strange place supposed to keep him safe,
Not even to smoke a B&H when he pleases.

Night 31: thinking about what I had witnessed during day 19.
Depriving one of their liberty so understanding of their
     situation seems immoral.

If the clinicians saw my thought process as the man had seen it
Would I likely experience the same treatment – detained under
     3 again?
Pulled away from my family without any notice – CTO revoked.
By day, I am professional, wading through the bureaucracy of
     services.
By night, I am deteriorating in mental state and body and no
     one notices.

The man, seemingly unwell and unkempt, noted that look in
     my eye.
His gaze instructed me not to let them win, to stay silent and
     pretend,
Or end up back in that place I despise – that we all despise.
I need help – I want to be helped, but I cannot return to that
     place.

The place where all doors are locked behind me out of fear,
And the doors remain closed for the same reason.

Herstory

Sarah Atayero

Blood-curdling screams, so loud I was momentarily deafened. Screams from a young woman that could have easily been me. Her beautiful, soft skin told a tale of self-loathing, hardship, and low self-esteem. As a woman, it's easy to imagine the difficulties in life that she's faced.

Some parts of her narrative remain a mystery. How did she end up here? The rolled-up sleeves of her jumper reveal old scars from self-mutilation on both lower arms, scars that lay next to newly pierced skin trying to heal. *I'm trying to heal.* These fresh cuts were not the source of her screams. It was the ice-cold needle being pressed into her buttock. It was the fact that she was being held, face down on a bed, by four mental health nurses – including myself. *This is not what I signed up for.* She continued to struggle. I pressed harder on her legs.

Two minutes earlier, everything had been calm – to an extent. As part of the response team, we'd been called to the female acute ward to help with an emergency. As I entered this woman's room, a senior nurse asked me and another nurse to comb through the woman's personal items to find any remaining shards of glass. Two male nurses restrained the woman's arms, and as they sat on the bed, one of the male nurses asked the woman what was going on? What had led her to smash a perfume bottle and attempt to use the glass to cut herself? 'Why are you doing this to yourself? You have so much potential.' Intermittently, the rest of the team chime in to add emotional support and affirmation for this distressed woman, trying to prevent the inevitable. 'Will you take your oral medication?' 'Please, please take your oral medication.'

'No.'

Screams. Screams so strong that I felt the vibration on my skin. Just like that, the situation changed from calm to hostile. It often ends like this, in a struggle. I'm beginning to understand why my first week as a support worker was spent learning different restraint techniques. 'This is for your own good, we're trying to help you.' *Am I helping?* Two injections to the butt, then we left to respond to another emergency. *I didn't sign up for this.*

Although, there's not always a struggle. A different patient who refused her oral medication was restrained so an injection could be administered. She didn't resist. She just lay there. She lay there while we gave her the injection, and she lay there when we left the room. I went back an hour later to check on her, and as I peered through the window to her room, she was still lying there – face down, not a single limb had moved. I called out her name to check she was still alive. 'Are you okay?'

'Yes.'

'Okay, well let me know if you need anything.'

'Okay.'

Then I left. *Am I helping?*

I remember my first day on the ward, standing in the nurses' station looking onto the communal area filled with patients. They're all mad. Completely and utterly mad. Of course, I didn't say this out loud: psychological training mixed with political correctness had taught me not to use such language. But I do remember thinking, surely no one could recover from this level of severe mental illness?

Four months in and I stand corrected. Some patients do recover, and it's a beautiful thing to see. It's a really fulfilling process to prepare a patient for discharge back to their home. It makes a fraction of the hard times worth it, that they are able to go home. *I hope I never see you again.* Sometimes I do see them again. The famously revolving door of mental health psychiatric inpatients.

In the time that I've worked on a female psychiatric intensive care unit, I've nursed thirty-five women. I could list them all by name – for obvious confidentiality reasons I won't. What I can say is that out of the thirty-five women, only eight were white, the rest were Black African or Black Caribbean. This shouldn't surprise you, this is a well-known and researched fact. In the UK, Black African and Black Caribbean individuals are 50 per cent more likely to be detained under the Mental Health Act via police referrals, restrained and forced to take medication. The only difference is that, *I'm now a part of that detention, restraint and injection.*

Situations like the ones described above were not in the job description when I applied. My naivety still stuns me. I have two degrees in psychology and I've been campaigning for better Black mental health treatment for the past few years. Yet every day when I go to work, I'm still in a state of disbelief regarding the distress Black patients that I care for experience. How did the system end up like this?

As both a psychology student and a mental health practitioner, I've been able to study mental health issues and observe them in practice. This has not been an easy road. A common emotion of mine is frustration. Frustration at the fact that mental health disorders, such as depression, are still thought of as 'white' issues. Frustration at the lack of research on the Black experience of mental health disorders. Frustration with an under-funded mental healthcare system where Black people fall through the cracks. Frustration that in order to change the system, I needed to become a part of it.

unpicking knowledge and power in mental health

Shuranjeet Singh

this is a short reflection on what i believe to be one of the most contentious, yet pressing issues facing the mental health landscape. it is something we can all provide, yet it is something that many of us are excluded from sharing. its meaning shifts continually, depending on what space you are navigating, and it is closely entangled within systemic processes of inclusion and exclusion. as such, when we share in one space we may be welcomed with open arms and our voices absorbed, but in others, our words may wash over confused minds like a stream over stones.

evidence

that is the word and concept i am going to begin to unpick today. it is something we have all been in contact with, however, its definition is often floating, where it is left up to the most dominant voices to take hold and shape what it 'really means'.

evidence is something used to 'make a case': whether it's to secure funding, to write an essay, to convey experiences and realities. evidence is a key component of how knowledge is constructed, knowledge which guides social, political, and economic decisions in our world.

here, i focus on traditional academic spaces. i don't look to critique or conform to particular measures, but to prompt the idea that evidence-making processes are temporal, contextual, and ultimately political. despite us wishing and hoping science to be neutral terrain, it is, in fact, riddled with processes informed by political, social, and economic agendas.

before presenting some thoughts on the place and politics of evidence in the mental health landscape, it is necessary to share a little about myself and how i found myself in this sector. through this context, my approach to evidence becomes clearly embedded in conversations around knowledge, power, and social justice.

me

having trained for four years as a social scientist, it became 'evident' (see what i did there?) that the ways in which we construct knowledge are not at all perfect and can, in fact, perpetuate as well as exacerbate latent social inequalities.

i particularly noticed this with research concerning punjabi and sikh communities where i could access information from a variety of sources: oral histories, conversations, objects, images, videos, as well as the more 'academic' papers and books. the in-depth discussions i had back home with family, friends, and local communities were vastly different to the realities presented in papers, which, despite being presented in the trappings of legitimacy, were perpetuating racist and reductionist stereotypes about my communities. there was an undeniable tension between the realities presented by academic and grassroots spaces.

i was soon introduced to the idea of discourse and how we 'make meaning' in our worlds. we all read the world through a framework, a complex tapestry that has been shaped by language, life experiences, and complex processes of socialisation. i recognised that there was more to 'knowing' than simply collecting, processing, analysing, and presenting information. critically appraising the information we gathered, the instruments used to process it, as well as challenging the nature of information itself was missing.

i then thought about how we structure and present knowledge. i started with broadsheet newspapers and the age-old 'times new roman' typeface. i then noticed peer-reviewed papers as the gold standard in academic worlds, the core building blocks of forming evidence in academic spaces which can be used to frame, uplift and critique arguments. as i slowly discovered, even across academic disciplines, there existed hierarchies of academic journals, methodologies, and university institutions themselves.

(de)mystifying mental health

the enlightenment in western europe is hailed as a seismic shift in scientific thought which prided itself on a perceived objectivity and rationality in relation to claims of divinity which had structured social hierarchies for so long. the legacies of the enlightenment exist in modern methodologies, the most reliable and robust of which are perceived as 'objective', that is, untouched by 'emotion' and 'bias'. a new terrain was formed for making evidence and knowledge claims which championed all that was perceived as objective, while looking down upon anything deemed subversive. while there are some advantages to the tools provided by the enlightenment, this period also provided the interpretive schema, a scientific justification, for subjugation and dehumanisation around the world.

it is well known that psychiatry and other medical disciplines emerged from industrialisation and slavery. the seventeenth and eighteenth centuries saw the onset of the industrial revolution in britain and other western nations, with wealth generated by ongoing colonial extraction and the transatlantic slave trade. concurrently, 'scientific' bases for racialised violence and dehumanisation manifested through eugenics and measures like skull shapes, also known as phrenology, which emphasised the inferiority of 'non-white races'. although such claims have since been dispelled, they highlight the contextualisation of 'evidence' and the weaponisation of science to perpetuate exclusion, extraction, and violence.

the mental health landscape is by no means power-neutral, and the quicker we acknowledge and understand that, the faster we can begin to confront and contest such challenges.

when i found myself in the mental health landscape, i quickly realised that the sector is driven forwards by different types of evidence. i recognised a number of different measures, frameworks, and tools which were championed. randomised controlled trials and PHQ-9/GAD-7 questionnaires stood out to me in my work in mental health academia alongside grassroots practice. more recently, experiential evidence through the involvement of those who have used mental health services or have lived experiences of mental health challenges offers another building block on how we construct knowledge, but it has been met with some hesitation.

time, money, methods

evidence-making is made possible through 'methods': processes by which evidential claims are framed as robust and reliable in a given context. the development of 'methods' evolve over time, but it is important to reflect on who, how, and why methods have emerged in mental health, as well as the context and capital required for constructing them.

reflecting upon existing methods, constructing a philosophical base for an alternative, and then building a framework that meets perceptions of robustness and reliability is no easy task. one of the most striking aspects of method-making is that it takes time and money to take them through rounds of testing, refinement, presentation, dissemination, and iteration. theoretically, no methodology is 'complete' and is constantly being improved through various avenues of academic intervention. generations of students, researchers, and academics contribute to developing methods. they do not appear overnight and require constant attention and watering, otherwise the academic landscape will swiftly move on to the next best thing. those methods which rise to the top become the gold standard, the preferred pathway by which evidence is made and ultimately, knowledge created.

how does our mental health landscape open space for those who are not afforded the time nor space to ponder, reflect and philosophise on how knowledge should be? the answer is that existing methodologies or philosophies have existed within marginalised communities for millennia. however, they have been actively pushed to the side, cast as 'irrational', 'unscientific' and even 'superstitious'. as such, methodologies and knowledge-making processes indigenous to racialised groups have been systematically erased, replaced, and those communities are now largely excluded from such discussions.

community-based solutions

within the context of the increasing marketisation of higher education as well as the structural and systemic barriers to entry within such spaces, those on the margins of society are placed further away from the academic and research conversations which concern them. a culture of exclusion not only removes their agency and voice from knowledge-making activities, but their experiences are taken through methodologies that have been created for them, not with them.

exclusionary ideologies permeate not only our politics and economy, but so too our academic institutions. the future, in my opinion, involves communities which are equipped to enquire, unpack, and develop solutions to their most pressing challenges. for this to be a reality, we must openly challenge the exclusion which permeates academic and research spaces, both in terms of workforce and within the toolkits used to devise evidence and make knowledge. it is a future where access to resources are responsive to need, whether academic, economic or social, to ensure that even those most marginalised within already excluded communities have access to the means of shaping knowledge and informing solutions.

organisations such as the participatory city foundation, chicago beyond, and the plethora of indigenous communities' research groups offer a framework through which we can turn exclusion into meaningful participation. within the mental health world, we require deep reflection and learning from those most affected by what we research. we need to work together not only to inform our study design but to shape methodologies, equalise recruitment, inform data governance, and manage effective dissemination as well as implementation.

the future of mental health research is focused on proximate localities, whether physical or even digital. the future of mental health research is fearless in contesting centuries of subjection, in demanding resources for change, and reclaiming the evidence and knowledge-making tools that have been so violently denounced.

He Was Treated Like a Criminal

Skye R. Tinevimbo Chirape

The impact of detention-related trauma on LGBTI+ refugees.

Introduction

Unlike other immigrants seeking asylum for reasons based on war, economic hardships, or political unrest, LGBTI+ persons often have been persecuted and disowned by family, society, culture, and religious communities. It means that when crossing international borders and claiming asylum, LGBTI+ persons seeking asylum often lack the support other refugees have. Following persecutory experiences in countries of origin, LGBTI+ persons seeking refuge may present with symptoms of psychological distress, but they face new challenges on reaching their destinations.

LGBTI+ individuals seeking asylum in the UK face prison-like conditions of detention, distressing legal asylum-seeking processes, and criminalisation by media rhetoric and immigration policy. The Home Office's practice of working on a system of *'disbelief'* and the difficulty in *'proving'* one's sexual orientation places LGBTI+ persons engaging with the asylum process at risk of detention in immigration removal centres. In addition to the process of waiting for a decision, a growing number of LGBTI+

claims are rejected, as the sexual orientation and gender identity of an applicant are disbelieved, landing applicants in immigration removal centres. Immigration removal centres also hold migrants and persons without British citizenship who have completed prison sentences for serious offences committed in the UK and are awaiting or contesting deportation. In addition, several prisons in the UK have been turned into Immigration Removal Centres. As a result, some of these detention centres are operated by HM Prison Service or private security contractors also outsourced to run prisons. This treatment of persons seeking asylum is influenced by the representations that link asylum directly to *'danger'*, risk and security issues; a discourse that permeates the popular media, political discourse, and policy statements.

'He was treated like a criminal'

This statement was extracted from an interview with a gay male-identifying refugee and represents the extent to which many LGBTI+ persons seeking asylum feel criminalised by the process of seeking asylum. Past research highlighting these challenges and my own experiences of seeking refuge were the catalysts for my study on how LGBTI+ persons seeking asylum construe their world. Specifically, my research sought to examine the personal constructs of a group of people that seek refuge in the UK on the basis of their sexual orientation and gender identification as this is a particular population that often experiences multiple facets of traumatic experiences (estrangement from culture, family and demands to prove sexual orientation). Accordingly, I interviewed seven adults who had been granted refugee status in the UK on the basis of their sexual orientation and gender identification, and two who were still in the process of seeking asylum on this basis. Below, I summarise a few of the constructs extracted from the experiences research participants shared with me during our conversations/interviews.

Injustice vs justice

All participants interviewed perceived that they had been treated unjustly and inhumanely. *'[It] feels like there is no justice when it comes to asylum seekers, especially for gay people,'* said one participant. This construct also expressed itself both through moral outrage towards injustice and acceptance or illusion that justice did not often occur. Participants showed a heightened awareness of justice. One individual reported that *'. . . feels bad . . . serves a purpose by speaking up, attending demonstrations,' '. . . always outspoken about it . . . attends demonstrations,'* and *'he fights every kind of injustices.'* Participants referred to ideas of justice or injustice with comparisons between their homeland and the UK. Equally, participants identified how this perceived injustice had a huge impact on their mental health.

Freedom vs restriction

Most participants recounted feelings of imprisonment, lack of control and of autonomy. Many referred to a sense of being restricted in movement. They communicated a desire to be *'free'* and be able to partake in various activities, events and/or take on opportunities. One person described that *'every human being deserves to be free, to be free to move, to express himself, . . . without fear of being detained'* and another account, *'. . . his life restricted by not having documents.'* Others described themselves as de facto prisoners, *'will feel like a prisoner . . . is restricted to a situation where she can't even go to the next town for a couple of days.'* When granted immigration status, participants describe feeling the freedom to 'go to work whenever, and I don't have to be scared when I go out, just in case you know the Home Office comes and pick me up. It's like I got more freedom' and freedom to 'try to get [on] with her life . . . freedom to travel, do whatever she wants to do . . . work and hobbies without feeling restricted.' In particular, participants reported how feelings of imprisonment continued to be present and have an effect on their mental health even after being given refugee status and perceptions of 'freedom'.

In limbo vs certainty

During the process of seeking asylum, both populations still in the process of seeking asylum and those granted refuge expressed feeling a sense of ambiguity regarding their future, '. . . didn't have status, where to live, know what he's doing tomorrow, what is happening the next day, the next week, the next month, the next year, . . . you are stateless, you don't have a status, you don't have a job, you don't have friends, you don't have anything, so he will be like a seaweed, just floating on sea.' Several individuals referred to experiencing a state of living in 'limbo' with an inability to move forward and make plans for the future, 'not being able to educate himself or have a decent job to make his life easier for him.' This appeared prevalent during the process of asylum-seeking as well as after being granted the status of refugee. A participant recounted experiencing shame and having to hide the fact that she did not have *legal* status to be in the UK.

Humiliation vs glorification/respect

The majority of those who participated in the research recounted experiences of feeling humiliation and shame, 'a time of humiliation . . . it was a time of humiliation . . . attitudes at the Home Office, the *people who make you sign on, they made you feel so small about yourself.'* They verbally revisited memories of situations that provoked feelings of humiliation, experiences of being devalued, disempowered and degraded, *'in [the] detention centre, it was awful. It was unbelievable . . . he was treated like a criminal . . . was stripped, left naked to move around . . . without eating . . . made him feel like he was a criminal . . . treatment was like you are not a human being, people talk to you like you are nothing'* and *'. . . was locked in a room with other strangers and had to knock and beg to be let out for the toilet . . . felt humiliated and discriminated against.'* Participants gave an account of how these experiences had profoundly affected their daily behaviour, both during the asylum-seeking process and after. Research contributors shared how, months following detention, they struggled to maintain a 'normal' life, experiencing anxiety, nightmares, panic attacks, and decreased self-worth and self-esteem. Others noted feeling fearful of re-engaging with society and described how this decline in mental health disrupted their ability to participate in other opportunities (i.e., employment, education, or social events) to help them develop.

Belonging vs not belonging

Several individuals expressed psychological concepts, including loneliness, alienation, and hopelessness, when reflecting a need to feel a sense of belonging. They expressed how they partook in particular activities to (re)gain a sense of community, a feeling of belongingness within a group, *'I go to groups with other people, different gay people.'* One individual, in particular, expressed the need to feel a sense of acceptance within the community, *'really wants to belong and be part of his community.'* Another individual communicated how she adapts herself to fit in and belong to a particular group of people, but also changes self to not offend others who may have different opinions about her sexuality. *'I'm going to people who are religious; I can't be going there looking all butchy . . . I kind of have to change me to fit other people.'* One person conveyed how, no matter the extent of the attempt to fit in and belong in British culture, he has continuously felt alienated and not accepted, *'[they] see me as not being part of this culture . . . because I am not culturally English. I still get asked where I come from . . . no matter how much I try to be British or no matter what I have done to contribute positively to the British identity, I still cannot be British.'*

Being in control vs not being in control

Individuals recounted situations which they felt diminished their personal sense of control and how these situations denied them happiness, *'I am never confident, I doubt myself every time, that's one thing I lack.'* They identified that their circumstances denied them employment and the right to further their education, which left them with feelings of not being in control, *'she can't work, she can't study, she can't even do anything without documents,'* *'she couldn't support the family, her partner and other people around her, couldn't even go to college.'* Many reported feeling anxious and not in control of their lives and daily events.

Conclusion

This study, which was part of an MSc in Forensic Psychology dissertation, was the first to evaluate the effect of detention-related trauma in LGBTI+ refugees. The research exposed refugees' consistent manner of construing self and the world around them to cope with detention and criminalisation by media and government control policies. Not only did the research outcome highlight the impact of the asylum-seeking process on the mental health of LGBT persons seeking asylum, but it also showed that a majority of individuals struggled to rebuild their lives under conditions of insecurity, uncertainty, and a decrease in mental health. Participants found it particularly difficult to make future plans. They expressed this uncertainty whether they were waiting for an outcome or had been granted UK asylum status. The uncertainty changed their view of self and their ability to live a 'normal' life.

The research highlights the impact of detention on an already vulnerable population. Participants perceived their situation as restrictive and disabling. The perceptions of losing free will and autonomy as a human is equated to mental defeat reported to occur when individuals experience helplessness, powerlessness, and uncontrollability.

A majority of participants described an acute sense of injustice. Each participant believed that a phase of their life had been irretrievably lost, due to detention and waiting for their application outcome. They felt that temporary visas denied future plans. One participant, in particular, reported that she has been hesitant to engage with employment opportunities for fear of discrimination. A majority described the *stateless person* and temporary visa period as weakening their sense of future control. Some recounted experiences in detention that cumulatively damaged their self-worth, including feeling criminalised by being detained in a prison-like environment and enduring multiple practices that seemed to them to be grossly unjust. The heightened alertness to injustice described by participants is akin to that described by those who have endured wrongful conviction and imprisonment. The research provided a compelling case for asylum policy and detention as having detrimental effects on the mental health of persons seeking asylum in the UK.

Postscript

When I first published this study, no other research had been undertaken regarding the personal constructs of LGBTI+ persons seeking asylum in the UK. Similarly, few studies had used a personal construct approach in cross-cultural studies. I am presently continuing this research at the University of Cape Town, where I am completing my Ph.D in Psychology, with the deliberate intention of adopting decolonial and feminist praxis for the research process. My thesis is provisionally entitled: *The Hare and the Baboon: Human (In)Security, migration and victimisation of African LGBT persons seeking asylum in the UK*. My recent article, 'Centring healing: reflexivity, activism and the decolonial act of researching communities existing on the margin' (2021), was published in the *Psychology in Society* (PINS) journal.

Words paint pictures, I'm an artist non-stop

David Sohanpal

How lonely can lonely be, is the world going crazy, or is it only me? Lonely isn't a strong enough adjective to describe all the nights that I've tried to grip tight and not lose my sanity. There are days where I am so depressed and a constant inner dialogue says, *just end this roller coaster ride you are on, I just want to slide into a hole where pain can't find me.* Should I be hanging on in quiet desperation, as is the English way? Do I follow my demons or take the path to be righteous?

How do I fight this? Meaning how do I write this . . . Hard as diamond, but I am in the ruff . . . the shortest straw has been pulled for me, I didn't deserve what was handed me. They ask why I seemed so solemn? As too many of us go to our graves with the song in our hearts left unwritten, will this be my swan song? Yeah, it's my life. It's my story, I have to put it to paper. They want the bright lights, but these are dark shadows. Enter my world of doom, consume fear and feel the panic . . . I am only trying to stay in the zone, with the right mindframe to survive this 'hostile environment'. Now let's go down the rabbit hole and view the world through my lens.

To be an asylum seeker in this great country . . . it is nothing like what you read in the tabloids, that we are given a big house, money, and life is rosy. I wish that was the case, my friend, but it is not true. In reality, you are trapped in this disarrayed, disfigured, impecunious world. Welcome to where time stands still.

Can't write about it all; there's no words that could describe the images in my head that visit me in my bed. Having been in silence for years while living in the shadows, poverty is one of the most malignant cancers. Being street homeless, not being able to get help because you have no recourse to public funds, even the council don't see you as a human being and will brush you off and say 'it is not our problem'.

I catch a panic attack, how can I calm down? Nervous that I might feel nervous, a vicious cycle. No one in my phone book I could call for assistance, they won't understand what I be goin through, what is this? Who can you turn to for help? Sometimes I look up at the stars and analyse the sky and ask myself, was I meant to be here?

I know this story too well; I can tell it with my eyes closed. Not sure you can stomach it? I have receipts made of scar tissue. It is living with a debilitating disease, a fish in an aquarium going in circles, the trauma paralyses you. Don't have anything to live for, not knowing where your next meal is coming from. You are stripped of all your rights, mentally shackled and the journey begins in an open-air prison for some, or in detention, and your mental health is going . . . is spiralling downwards. They throw us in a jail that is operated like a zoo.

Most people who have come here have already suffered a significant amount of trauma; seeing your whole family executed in front of you or beaten to a pulp because of your beliefs. I have been through all kinds of hate and pain, hard to feel at home here in this body that my trauma lives in.

Only the mirror knows my pain and my tribulations! Didn't have a pot to piss in, and for real, how does it feel to have to stretch a fiver to last a week? What do you know about getting moved from place to place and sleeping in the cold below freezing or spat on while you sleep? Waking up is a struggle, I start feeling dizzy, and now my heart's beating out of my chest. It's happening again, it's happening again, but you can't tell nobody, they goin to think you crazy.

I am only reminding you of things that you already know.

I have been asked countless times – how do I cope with it, how do I deal with it? To be honest I don't have a simple answer, but I have to give a shout out to my solicitor Georgina, aka 'The World's Best Solicitor', who believed in me even when I didn't, when I was down in the darkest place, she went above and beyond. I was ready to press that self-destruct button cause I had lost faith in the immigration system, and I'd given up on solicitors who had been fleecing me. I was ready to quit, and I threw my hands up at the world to say, 'fuck it'.

No one understood me except for my solicitor, so thank you for not brushing me away like the others did, even when you didn't have the capacity. I am not sure if she remembers the first time we spoke when I called the helpline; we spoke for about forty-five minutes; I instantly felt the compassion and sincerity in her tone of voice that reassured me things will be okay. For the first time in my life, I had a real solicitor, someone who cares, who listened even when I was being adamant and who didn't stop me abruptly halfway through just to let me know what their hourly rate was. I had to pinch myself to see if I was dreaming or if this was real, have all the stars aligned or what? It makes a big difference when someone actually believes in you and treats you with dignity like a human being, I felt it was like a godsend or fate; a big sister looking out for a little bro who had gone astray.

Look at us now, all that we've been through.

I have always found nature comforting, calming and a great form of escapism. I became street homeless around October

2019, and when the lockdown came it was surreal, like a post-apocalyptic film. I walked everywhere, there was no traffic or noise pollution and the city was deserted. Even the foxes would come out in the daytime.

The only people you would see in the streets were homeless people; they had nowhere to go, they couldn't self-isolate; as all shelter, day centres and coffee shops were closed. We were left on the streets. The animals found there was less food, and it was the same for us, as few charities would come out to hand out food.

I used to seek refuge in the parks and spent hours just sitting and watching the birds, squirrels coming up to you. The night was quiet, and I could hear the foxes' vocalisations. I would always take some food for them, and sometimes they would come right up to me when I was sleeping. My wake-up call was the chorus of birdsong, pigeons cooing and squirrels chasing each other in the trees. When it rained I couldn't leave any food out, so in the morning they would come find me to let me know it was time for breakfast.

When it rained, you could smell and taste it, as if you were back in the bush. I would brush my teeth with the rainwater. I used to cycle along the canal where I would feed the geese and a family of swans every morning. The swan had four babies who would hop on her back while they were travelling. I wondered, how many babies can she fit? Each week I would see them change; growing slightly bigger and slowly changing colour. When I did not see the swan, I did wonder, where did they go? If they went up the canal, I hoped I would see them on my way back.

I would paint in the park, which was a great distraction from my anxiety, and leave it to dry overnight. Art therapy allows expression of traumatic experiences without the use of words. When I paint or draw I felt I had regained my freedom, my autonomy, I could draw/paint anything, anytime and anywhere. No one told me what to do or how to do it; I just went with the flow.

Painting in this tiny hotel room is difficult; paint goes all over the walls, carpet and everywhere. I feel like a caged animal, as if someone had clipped my wings even before I could fly. I wish one day I could have my own garden so I can paint and observe the wildlife while listening to their songs.

Since I was given a hotel room by the Home Office, I feel like I am in a prison. During the hot weather, it was really difficult . . . if I closed the window to avoid the construction noise there would be no air. I couldn't breathe, I feel like I am suffocating.

When I was homeless, I was happy being out with Mother Nature, sleeping under a tree surrounded by foxes and waking up to the sounds of wildlife, the morning dew on my sleeping bag, the breeze blowing in my face. There was always fresh air, even when it was below freezing.

Now, I try to spend most of my time at a local park lying on the grass, drawing, feeding the swan and the ducklings. Recently, I fed a few crows, and a few days later, I was surrounded by a few more. I think one of them told the rest where to get food . . .

I want to tell people I am not here to steal your jobs or destroy your culture, I want to stand on my own two feet and not depend on any charity. I can learn from you as you can learn from me, I would like to be like you, to help my community, pay tax and be safe. A paper doesn't define me; I am still the same person that left my birth country. I did not suddenly grow two horns or become a criminal because I am seeking protection.

Besides art, I enjoy donating blood as, in my own small way, I know I am giving back to the community. It makes me feel like a person with a purpose in life, even if it was only for a few short minutes. One day while donating blood, I asked the nurse what is this 'NEO' marked on my card. She told me your blood is not stored in the blood bank and it is to be used for new-born babies as you didn't have any disease when you were young – you are special. Newborn babies can only be transfused with blood that lacks the cytomegalovirus, and my blood is CMV-negative. Now if my blood saves your child's life, would you look at me with new eyes and call me your brother or would you still ask me to go back home, immigrant?

I consider myself lucky to have met some lovely people from LJAG, New Art Studio, SanteProject, Refugee Council, NNLS and lovely Georgina and JCWI who have helped me, supported me and shown me I am someone. I am a valued member of their community even if the state doesn't see that yet!!!

When I was street homeless, New Art Studio was my first home. New Art Studio is family, the family that I never had and always wanted. So thank you Tania, Ruanna and Jasmin for being real and keeping it real, real teachers teach real things!! It is still a way to escape for a few hours and to spend time doing what I love, making art, which feels like magic from a blank canvas. You pour out all your emotions on it and it becomes something beautiful. Even just sharing a cup of tea with people who have similar experiences of anxiety and trauma feels like a relief, free from any judgements. Humans learnt to draw before we could speak: from the evidence of all those cave paintings we were visual people, but have lost it along the way.

We all have powers, it's not mystical, but you have power; you might have the power to comfort somebody with your words, or with your presence. Sometimes we need to plant seeds; sometimes we need to pull weeds.

I'm thinking of ending things

Vee

I am so burnt out.

I once had a mentor who told me that it was important that I didn't share my weakest moments with the world because it delegitimises my business capabilities. Instead of protecting me, this advice simply made my burdens harder to bear, fuelling the underlying issue: people's failure to see me as someone capable of vulnerability. What is more human than the desire to be understood? And how will anyone ever understand if I am afraid to share what I am going through?

My community work is primarily based on mental health and providing members of my community respite from their day-to-day stresses. This work was born out of my struggles with my own mental health, having had a breakdown when I was twenty-one.

I remember it like yesterday. I showed up half in outside clothes, half-pyjamas. I hadn't washed in days. I hadn't had a hot meal in four weeks. I hadn't slept for more than four hours a night in two weeks. I got a first in the exam.

Once I was on antidepressants and sleeping pills and considering if I should actually take my antipsychotic medicine ('I'm not crazy!!'), I knew that no one should have ever been in my position.

I felt that I had done everything 'right' and sought help, yet, here I was.

My mental health decline was triggered by a violent sexual assault during my first year of uni. I was absolutely broken up, and worse still, I had no one. No one knew something was wrong, no one noticed that I had gone missing, no one noticed self-harm scars or the destructive and reckless behaviours that ensued. I knew I was out of control. I went to women's crisis centres, university counselling, disclosed my assault to my university so that I could get help. I did the *things*. So why couldn't I get over it? Why did I still have a breakdown?

Largely, they were not equipped to deal with my issues. It was always, 'Why don't you talk to your parents about how you're feeling?' *For them to ask me how I can be depressed with a roof over my head, food in my belly and clothes on my back?*

Things began to change when I discovered camping. There was a low buzz of excited but peaceful conversation as the girls and I huddled in for the night to connect. There was no wind; we didn't need it for the abundance of fresh air where we were sleeping that night. I remember feeling so small and like all of my problems were not really problems because the world was so vast. My experiences were not part of the karmic equation that needed to be balanced; nature is not evil. If I am in nature, I am *safe* because even if I get hurt, nothing was trying to hurt me with evil intentions. I'm not saying that nature can't be hard to accept sometimes, but I am saying that the reason that a falcon eats a cute bunny rabbit isn't that it hates it; it's because food fi get nyam.

The camping trip was liberating. The only reason I was there was to get away from the UK and far away from where I had suffered. It felt like I had taken such a horrific experience, and I had made something beautiful out of it. Never in my life had my problems felt so manageable as they did when I tilted my head back to look at the stars. Living white balls, battling the embrace of an inky black sky. It didn't terrify me; it validated that the universe was expansive, and I was here, and here was perfect, so everything else must be perfect. It must be exactly as it is supposed to be.

Being a survivor is no Medal of Valour. Most days, it feels like drowning in a river and only having just enough oxygen for your legs to keep pushing against the current. Leading up to my breakdown, I became cruel, pointed, emotionally volatile. I lost whole days, experiences, conversations that I can't remember and probably never will. And while this loss was tragic, I had almost been gifted with a new compassion for survivors of gendered violence. After a whole month of making friends with women and later learning of similar violent experiences, I mentioned to a friend, 'survivors always find me'. Perhaps, I sought them out too, to share the burden that I couldn't when I locked myself away for several weeks when I was nineteen. Who else would know the feeling of having your soul snatched from you by someone who absolutely disgusts you? Who else would know what it's like to be in transition from childhood and not only think of ways to hurt yourself but ways to destroy yourself completely? Who else would know what it's like to sit in your room on New Year's Eve, listening to everyone scream in the sounds of the new year and all the new beginnings, hoping someone would notice that you wouldn't be moving on with them all?

> Captive Maternals are self-identified female, male, trans or ungendered persons feminized and socialized into caretaking within the legacy of racism and US democracy.
>
> – Joy James

As a descendent of enslaved people, I can relate.

The state had refused to take care of me until I was at breaking point, used medication as some kind of *band-aid on a bullet hole* **after** my trauma turned into a crisis and then made me wait 800+ days for psychotherapy on the NHS. Three years from asking for help to receiving the help I needed. In that time, I experienced a thousand petty humiliations, the worst for me being period poverty and medication poverty.

This is why, as part of my community work, I asked members to donate sanitary products to food banks. I could think of nothing worse than being unable to feed your family and then getting the dreaded cramp that signals that your period is coming. Poverty robs you of choices, and I knew too many people who have experienced period poverty, who opted to take contraceptives to prevent or reduce the bleeding. Irrespective of whether poor people with periods hate their periods or not, they should have options.

> Captive Maternals are designated for consumption in the tradition of chattel slavery; they stabilize with their labor the very social and state structures which prey upon them.
>
> – Joy James

Is this what I had been doing? Stabilising the labour of the very state structures that harmed me by designing this space? Was I relieving the state of its responsibility to the communities I was serving by doing their job for them?

My team *was* tired. They had all dedicated somewhere between two months and two years working on this project. And I mean they really dedicated themselves to it. From one of them driving dozens of miles to collect equipment to another prepping several projects only for them to be shut down by government lockdowns and flaky advice. Racism, sexism, homophobia, trans-phobia, islamophobia, ableism and immigration are just a **few** of the things that my team struggle with – on top of managing their *own* mental health during this time.

Some days it felt like we were being forced to compromise our kindness and compassion in order to get the job done. Planning outdoor events is no easy task, as you have to factor in things like on-site security and rain (lol). Still, we were determined. When someone fell off, we quickly regrouped to pick things back up again.

But I'm tired.

And they're tired.

And we deserve to rest.

We deserve to have someone to look at our faces, to know that we're tired and that we're doing our best. We're now frequently being mistaken for a corporation that is trying to make big bank – folks think I want to capitalise off my own trauma.

No doubt, there's a lot to think about. And I'm spending a lot of time doing it.

I realised that in sharing the burden of this very difficult community work (and when I say burden, I don't mean it in its truest sense, I mean it the same way a parent might feel about a child), I had turned my team into people who others were incapable of seeing as vulnerable. And they are vulnerable; we all are. They are the roots of the community, spreading under the earth and holding us up; people who saw an issue, believed in my vision for a solution and stepped up to pull it off. I want them to be able to go to work and feel safe, comfortable, like they can be themselves and never, ever burn out.

I want their vulnerability to be acknowledged, their mental health protected. I want them to be able to do this work without it sapping their vitality before their labour collapses with a bang or a whimper.

I want this for myself too.

I don't know what to say beyond this, because . . . I was only *thinking* about ending things.

Indigo

And there are times we see in indigo. Mood indigo,
through murky waters and looming shadows.

Mind the Gap

Hana Riaz

One

At 7.20 a.m. on the furthest end of the Northern Line platform at Clapham Common, a woman falls onto the tracks as the Tube approaches. She does not realise she is falling until the weight of the train is against her.

The driver says he didn't see her.

A spectator says they didn't see anybody push her.

Another witness says they don't think she tripped. In fact, they are sure she hadn't.

Two

Every day, Saliha is used to meeting patients that tell her that they are in pain because they are not not in pain. The absence of pain becomes the measurement of whether pain is really a thing that is happening to the body. This time, she's in the patient's bed, trying to listen out for it.

As her eyes flutter open, her vision is soft and hazy. Javed is standing next to the bed holding a cup, her mum just a fraction behind him. A strange mix of Dettol and burnt coffee lingers in the room.

'Babe, how you feeling? Don't try to move too much.'

Her mother abruptly interrupts him:

'Betti, are you in pain?'

A doctor walks in and asks the same question.

'Where does it hurt? On a scale from one to ten, how painful is it?'

Three

For the last ten months, Saliha has been treating a patient everyone else on the ward has now lost interest in. Maya has just turned sixteen and claims she is in love. Routinely, she came in with black and indigo bruises. Sometimes, she needed stitches.

Even then, Maya is the type of understated pretty that people know how to take advantage of, and this makes Saliha protective of her. Saliha never probes too much during Maya's visits, knowing full and well that teenagers will all too often retreat and do the opposite of what an adult tells them to do. She learns to fight the motherly instinct she believed was buried so deeply it ought to be dead.

'I hope you're not missing school because of this,' she'd say to Maya, drawing the curtain shut.

Four

Saliha tries to remember the moment before she hits the train but is afraid to. She tries to recall if there was anything different about that morning. She attempts to start from the beginning but always skips the part about feeling. There was something less accurate about trying to remember feelings. Instead, she was almost superstitious with routine; routine was a reliable set of acts that could be remembered.

Saliha is a morning kind of person, her husband Javed is not. Javed is heavy-handed with everything, always manages to roll over to her side of the bed and displace her. Leaves a trail of everything he does everywhere he goes. She hates this. Has to be neat and compact. Javed that day was on her side of the bed when they woke up, watching her through the sleep in his eyes.

She remembers the walk to the station, remembers eating an apple that was soft and bruised and unsweet. She remembers the autumn leaves that were probably beautiful only a few days before, ground into slippery mounds on the pathway. She remembers carrying a photograph of her daughter in her wallet and taking it out only when she had left the house.

Five

When Saliha bought her first house, she renovated the garden immediately. The peeling paint in the hallway was less important than the right number of magnolia trees ready to bloom in spring.

She hired a company called Javed & Co. and was surprised to find Javed & Co. was really just Javed – a tall, broad-shouldered guy in his early thirties who looked messy but was strangely meticulous and particular when she showed him what she wanted to be done. He ignored all her ideas, told her to trust him. She almost wanted to say no – no one had ever tried to change her mind about anything before – but she gave in.

When the garden was completed, Javed and Saliha stood at the kitchen window, steaming cups of coffee in hand, staring at what once seemed wasted and sad turn ordered and beautiful.

He asked how she knew all the names of all the plants, even the ones she hadn't asked for. Saliha explained she was a bit like a hand-me-down daughter; her mother passed down everything she learnt, including the botany she studied at school in Pakistan. She thought it was an important thing to be able to name and classify, like naming gave objects a deliberate purpose in the world even if it was just to be beautiful.

Javed picked up the empty cups from the countertop and began to wash them. For a moment, she imagined her mother visiting her new home, rearranging everything she had decorated. She felt a sudden sense of relief in trusting him with the garden.

Six

When Javed leaves the room to get them tea, Saliha's mother finally breaks the silence.

'Did you see who did it; who pushed you? The CCTV footage was fuzzy. If you remember what they look like, we can see if they can trace it on the other cameras. I want us to sue them. Of course, Javed won't want to do any such thing, but I want to make sure someone pays for this!'

Saliha doesn't respond, instead wishing there were windows to look out onto the hospital courtyard.

Seven

The last time Saliha saw Maya, she was sitting at the edge of the hospital bed swinging her legs.

'Can I go now, doc?' Maya asked.

'Did you know you're pregnant?'

Maya shrugged.

'Well, you are. Six weeks or so.'

'Do you have any kids, doc?'

'I did . . . I mean, I do.'

'Girl or boy? How old are they?'

'Ten. A girl. You know you have options; if you'd like, I can talk you through them . . . are you going to tell your boyfriend? Will you be safe?'

'I don't mean to be rude, but I've gotta go. My aunt will get suspicious if I'm not home on time.' Maya hopped off the bed, grabbing her school rucksack from the side table as she left.

Eight

A few weeks before the accident, Javed took Saliha to a place on the coast that was a few hours away from London. Even though it was spring, it stormed the entire weekend. Craving the salt on her skin, she took long walks alone on the beach anyway, and watched the sand sink further into the ground after each step.

At some point, she remembered her first year of medical school, falling pregnant with just enough time to hide it. She remembered hiding the pregnancy, failing the year, leaving her boyfriend, the feeling of an unknown thing taking her body hostage. How lonely the lies were, how cold and long the winter was up in that part of the country, throwing out old clothes that no longer fit, feet that ached and ached, the library she couldn't escape, the nausea that would force itself in the middle of a class, the wrong answers, how – to feel less lonely – she learnt to speak in a quiet voice to the thing taking her body hostage. How uncontrollable the process was, how easy the lies became, how unbearable it was anticipating an indefinite loss. The end of the summer arrived, and with it giving the baby up to a couple she believed she could trust. She asked only one thing of the adoptive parents: to keep the baby name she had carefully chosen. Ready to move back to London, she packed away her things with all the secrets.

Nine

The morning of the accident, Saliha was haphazard in the shower and cut her skin with the razor. She rushed and stained the towel. Javed was still asleep on the wrong side of the bed. She looked at him, his face sombre but tender with love. On the way to the station, she ate an apple that was soft and bruised and unsweet, an autumn leaf caught on the bottom of her shoe, her image distorted in the mirrors at the Tube entrance, and she frowned in its place. She put her daughter's picture back into her wallet. It was no more crowded than it ever is at 7.20 a.m. on the furthest end of the Northern Line platform at Clapham Common. At that exact moment, she thinks of Maya and observes the pain before it leaves so fleetingly.

Ten

Saliha is in and out of things when Maya appears the next morning, standing at the edge of her hospital bed.

'Heard you jumped in front of a train, doc,' her voice absolute in the way only children dare name a thing so directly. 'I wanted to tell you I left him; I finally left him. Can you believe it?'

'Sounds like a fresh start.'

Saliha smiles, small but sweet as Maya rests her hands on hers. She imagines the magnolia trees in her garden in bloom, the struggle of winter returning and finally left behind.

Plea in the Dead of Night

Niki M. Igbaroola

I want to write about my pain.

About how hurt saw me and made a dive for the unfilled parts
of my heart, setting up home and hearth.

I want to write about the tears behind these eyes, clear as I
furiously type this out. Torrent helmed by part-exhaustion,
part-screaming grief.

About the guilt I feel for going so many months without sitting
with God.

About the rage and pain that have kept me a cautious distance
from him.

I want to make him stop it – life, the uncertainty.

The cycle that is causing more dizziness than I bargained for.

This is enough, it has to be.

I am broken so much on the inside, I fail to recognise the
woman on the out.

I have fragments floating about inside me, sending tiny
shockwaves every second, so I never forget that wholeness
departed this vessel several stops ago, with a relieved sigh
and an optimistic smile.

This body is alien.

I see glimpses of me sometimes, but for the most part, it's like
    being trapped in a body belonging more to another:
GET OUT!

I want to yell at the me looking in on shattered me:
'Come out and join the rest of us,' but my mouth is too worn
    down by weariness to form words.
I can't see a way out.
Sleep is little relief, because tomorrow always comes.
It has its needs and wants and desires, and is seductive in its
    demands, adamant that they be met.
I cannot say no to tomorrow – she is vicious in her tenacity;
She bites and nips and snarls at my heels.
I am never quick enough nor ready enough for her.
How someone so full can have such little time in her baffles me.
Brain half-aware of what is really going on.

I can't cry anymore. It's too sad.
I'm too sad.
But the need to cry is choking me.
Holding me hostage in my own body.
Face squeezed tight in an effort to cry/subdue my impending
    tears.
Who can tell? Save me. Somebody.

Save me, if you can hear me.
End the madness without and within.

when you can't sleep

Esme Allman

She stirs as you watch on from across your bed. A snore escapes her, rumbling in her nose. You place your hand on her back, rubbing circles to silence her, restoring a peaceful sleep. You turn yourself onto your side, pushing your weight into your hands and manoeuvre yourself to face outwards, towards the room; careful not to wake your sleeping friend. The mirror placed on the wardrobe opposite reflects the dull shapes in the 4 a.m. darkness. It's no use trying to sleep now. The buzz from the evening before has worn off, but your friend is now in her fifth hour of sleep, her eyes fluttering depths of slumber, a murmur loosens her lips every so often. You replay the evening in your head:

A wander across a bridge. A sun setting into a brilliant blue and pink, an orange creeping in. A route you've taken for years, sat up on that hill overlooking a separate part of the city. Lighter. Spark. Exhale. Dull.

Everything moving slow. Your friend lost in a fit of giggles, and you too, laughing at her laughter. A sound escapes the hole in her face right from the pit of her stomach. She's rolling on the grass at one point, and you smile at this child-like woman amid something endearing. It's disarming. There's a brightness to her in the middle of the dusk, soon to be followed by a night gently setting in. Your head is lolling, and you consider when you'll slip back into darkness again.

The sun begins to crawl into the sky, blurring night and

morning into eerie dawn. It's seldom you sleep on nights like these. You feel it creep up on you; special moments when you remember you are, in fact, alive turned insignificant and mundane. At midnight you stared through the darkness at your reflection, praying for rest. At one, your reflection looked back at you from a hopeful distance. At two, you stopped fighting. By three, your thoughts had gained some momentum, whizzing with an easy menace around your head. They chase each other, heavy and sticky.

You eye a photograph of yourself that leans against a row of books, remembering how the young girl stood in them used to be. Lighter. Happier. A mouth that beamed. Two crinkled dimples on each cheek. A crease in your forehead when something like joy erupted from you. Cheeks bloated from smiling so excessively. A draught moves its way through the space, sending a shiver across the room. The photograph slips from its careful position and skids its way to the floor by the foot of your bed. The little girl looks back at you, now upside down, not smiling, now grimacing. You mouth something to her. Maybe *Hello*. Maybe *Sorry*. It's no use. Your pulse, now waterborne, the ripple within your body gripping you.

As you begin to feel yourself fall, you look to your friend, her knees tucked into her body, cradling herself in her sleep. You remember her hand against your cheek a few hours prior. A cool pulse of something radiating against your face. She kisses your forehead, tells you how much she missed you and how good it is to have you back. Standing between the abyss of her and her words, her hand, her kiss. You stare blankly into it. Nothingness behind you. Toes curled over its edge, undecided on your fight-or-flight ultimatum. You seat yourself on the edge, let your legs dangle idly and continue to stare. You make out the figure of your friend on the other side. The vague colours of a sunset. Smoke. Surrounded by more nothingness.

You stay on its edge. And your friend sleeps. You feel a wave of blue roll its way up your body, pulsating through. It feels weird to be so awakened by this thing. This thing that makes you retreat into yourself for weeks, months. The thing that makes a home out of your resistance. That hollows out your eyes from sleeplessness. The one that forces words to disintegrate from your throat when asked if you're okay. The one that silences that beg, that whimper to reach out to your friend, who lies across from you, and just tell her. Tell her everything.

She stirs, louder this time. Lets out a moaning stretch and speaks into the opposite wall. 'You awake?'

'Go back to sleep,' you say. 'It's not morning yet.'

Cassen Awa*

Raman Mundair

Exhausted, tender, cradle
head in hands. Dry
scalp offers snow,
fingers comb
     feathers
     of hair fall
something leaves
offerings to the thin day
baptised with tears.

---

* *Cassen Awa* – Shetland dialect for something that is shed, sacrificed.

Depression, Doubt, and Deliverance

Ololade A.

'When a stranger sojourns with you in your land, you shall not do him wrong. You shall treat the stranger who sojourns with you as the native among you, and you shall love him as yourself, for you were strangers in the land of Egypt: I am the LORD your God.'
Leviticus 19:33–34

Being the child of immigrants has undoubtedly shaped my self-perceptions and mental health experiences. In the late eighties, my Nigerian parents migrated from the motherland to peculiar, foreign soil. In their newfound adulthood and freedom, they saw opportunities and worked hard to make a living through low-paid, odd jobs – cleaning, cabbing, security – whatever they could get their hands on to survive. Far from being unique, these sentiments are echoed through the many stories and experiences in our communities.

Many of our parents eventually left the hustle of their younger years and managed to get stable nine-to-fives, only to be overlooked for promotions. Meanwhile, their white colleagues, sometimes junior staff who they had mentored, seamlessly rose through the ranks, leaving them in the dust. Our parents have tried their best to assimilate, yet have never quite managed to fit in or blend in with the crowd. Our parents are somewhat content with the lives they have built here and the legacy they've passed on through their children; yet, somewhere, in the back of their minds, they long for home.

These first-generation diasporans take pride in their experiences: hardship and survival back home growing up, followed by resilience and survival here. They developed invaluable transferable skills and adapted accordingly. All over the world, Black people have routinely beat the odds of failure. From generation to generation, we survive and resist various forms of oppression. Afro Caribbean immigrants and their descendents have become adept at surviving – and often excelling – in the face of routine discrimination and institutionalised racism.

However, our collective strength can also be a thorn in our side. A tough-love attitude manifests through the brushing off of complaints. We just get on with it like we always have, whatever 'it' is. A mindset persists that your Goliath isn't as bad as you're making it out to be. We shall overcome, right? Fears and anxieties threatening to swallow you whole get dismissed by elders who barely bat an eyelid. Cue ever-so-subtle victim-blaming. They tell us our worries are unfounded, that our generation's lives are easy, that we should be happy and grateful.

'Your generation is weak and doesn't know hardship.'

'If you've never had it bad, then you won't know what good is.'

Even among our peers, instead of admitting we are at breaking point, we often tend to 'firm it' and suffer in silence.

These pervasive attitudes make it very difficult to admit that you're struggling with mental health issues, let alone seek help for them. Tough love causes us to bury our heads in the sand. In the UK, Black people are four times more likely to be detained under the Mental Health Act than white people. Detention is often used as a last resort and in moments of acute crisis. We miss the warning signs and access mental health services in traumatic circumstances, which ends up being more of a hindrance than a help. In my personal experience, a Black person admitting they are seeing a therapist is often viewed with incredulity or suspicion rather than bravery or as a radical act of self-care.

There are many factors that shape our attitudes to mental health. Many Black people are raised in Christian households. In Pentecostal and Evangelical strands, there is a particularly strong emphasis on faith healing and the belief that many issues can be cured with prayer. Being depressed and anxious may be viewed, at best, as symptomatic of a lack of faith and an ungrateful spirit. At worst, they are attributed to demonic possession.

Regardless of your views on the supernatural realm, this can have serious social and psychological consequences for affected individuals and their families. A person in the throes of a psychotic episode may be viewed with fear by their wider communities, or shunned altogether, with long-lasting damage. This may take the form of ruined reputations, shattered self-esteem, difficulty in maintaining relationships and poorer health outcomes in the long term.

'Hear my prayer, LORD;
let my cry for help come to you.
Do not hide your face from me
when I am in distress.
Turn your ear to me;
when I call, answer me quickly.'
Psalm 102:1–2

'The Lord is close to the brokenhearted and saves those who are
crushed in spirit. The righteous person may have many troubles,
but the Lord delivers him from them all'
Psalm 34:18–19

As a child, I always had my head buried in a book, and I am still a voracious reader to this day. However, hindsight has made me realise that my love for fiction was deeper than a love for the characters within the pages; it was an unhealthy form of escapism . . . During my teenage years, I wrestled with serious bouts of anxiety and depression, but it was not until my final year of university that I recognised my experiences for what they were.

It was in my final year of university that the bomb detonated. The trigger? A relationship breakdown, compounded by isolation, university stress, low self-esteem, repressed issues from my childhood, and doubts about my Christian faith. For the first time in my life, I recognised that I was incredibly hurt and angry. Furious. A switch had been flicked on.

Looking back, the signs had been there for a couple of years. Despite being moderately active and health-conscious, I always felt exhausted. However, I had convinced myself it was mostly physical. If I exercised more, took supplements, ate a better diet, had a better attitude, and stopped questioning God all the time, I would be fine. How could I not expect to be slow and tired with all the excess weight I was carrying? I was the common denominator, right?

It did not help that these sentiments were echoed by my well-intentioned parents. I just needed to be a little bit more consistent and organised, think positively and try harder. However, the fatigue persisted, and I started to wonder if this was an issue of the mind, rather than a purely physiological one.

'Am I tired because I'm lazy? Or am I lazy because I'm tired?'

Questions like these popped up in my head every so often, but I ignored them and carried on as normal. Blood tests at the GP didn't flag up any abnormalities.

'All clear, nothing to worry about – you're normal!'

Then in my final year, things got really bad. I was tearful all the time, crying constantly but hiding it very well in public. I was triggered by the tiniest things. I could be sitting in a lecture absentmindedly, driving home for the weekend or laughing with a friend; then suddenly, my mood would shift. A dark cloud would overcome me, then tears. I vividly remember once, after a lecture, I went into a toilet cubicle and did my usual routine of silent weeping. Shortly after, a friend came into the loo, so I instantly stopped crying, wiped my face, flushed the toilet and exited the cubicle with a huge smile plastered on my face. She didn't suspect anything.

No matter what I did, there always seemed to be an underlying sadness I couldn't shake, and it would come out at the most inopportune moments. The brain fog was unshakeable. I struggled to concentrate on course assignments and reading straightforward articles. I tried really hard, but I just could not seem to focus on anything. I had insomnia at night and slept most of the day. When I went home on the weekends, all I seemed to do was eat, sleep, and stay in my room. I isolated myself and stopped making an effort with my appearance. My parents knew something was up, but they could not figure out what it was.

During sleepless nights, I would leave my flat, get into my car and drive down long, winding, black country roads. Depression turned it from a therapeutic hobby into a twisted pastime. I wasn't actively facilitating my death, but I was very reckless, doing ridiculous speeds in pitch-black, narrow country lanes, vaguely hoping that I would round a corner, hit a deer at full speed, and be killed instantly. That was one of my recurring fantasies. I was too scared to take my own life, but I passively wanted to die through other means. Once, on the way to seeing a friend, I stood on a Tube platform, and an overwhelming urge to jump came over me. I reined it in and continued my journey.

By April of the following year, I knew I needed to get help. I did an online screening for depression on the NHS website and scored 24 out of 27. With the encouragement of a close friend who was being treated for depression, I eventually went to my local GP. Explaining my symptoms, he diagnosed me with moderate depression. I was not surprised at all. That day, instead of shame and condemnation, I felt relief. It was not all in my head, nor was it something that could easily be cured with yoga and listening to worship music. It was real.

I would not tell my parents for another month or so, and when I did, they were horrified. At the time, I felt like they were more concerned about the diagnosis being on my medical record than what was going on inside my head (although their reactions were more out of shock than callousness). They were worried that I had blighted my chances of getting a good job and that the stigma of mental health had all but eliminated the chances of me marrying a fellow African. Taking antidepressants was also a major concern. Those initial conversations we had were very tense, but I was in no doubt that my wellbeing was their primary concern. On the whole, they were, and continue to be, my biggest supporters.

'I waited patiently for the LORD;
he inclined to me and heard my cry.
He drew me up from the pit of destruction,
out of the miry bog,
and set my feet upon a rock,
making my steps secure.'
Psalm 40:1–2

I gradually regained my self-confidence and stabilised. Nearly three years later, I maintain that treating depression holistically – through support from family and friends, medical treatment, talking therapies, rediscovering and embracing my faith for myself – drastically improved my outcomes. They have helped me to not only survive and stay afloat but to thrive.

I have a strong support system through family, church, and my wider social circle. There are a number of people I talk to about my concerns who are supportive and non-judgemental. When you are feeling low, you don't always want a rousing speech or quick-fix solution; you just want to know people love you enough to patiently sit in that space with you until you feel better again.

I no longer take antidepressants; however, I would never discourage anyone who takes them from doing so. For many people, a stable medication regime and a good psychiatrist are literally life-savers. One of Jesus' apostles, Luke, is described in the New Testament as a physician. Medical intervention and faith are not mutually exclusive – on the contrary, they complement one another. To presume otherwise would be extremely ignorant.

Nowadays, I experience the occasional dip, but on the whole, I have learned to not be too hard on myself. My faith has also played a huge role in my recovery. In life, there are undoubtedly moments for joy, laughter, and ecstatic praise. However, there were also times in the Bible where people such as David in the Psalms and Job prayed for God to end their lives in moments of utter despair. God promises to be with us and to comfort us in times of suffering, not to prevent suffering altogether.

We need to change attitudes in our communities towards mental health. Instead of demonising people who are struggling, or seeing them as weak, there is an alternative. We can use ancestral resilience, community support, and spirituality, coupled with modern medical and therapeutic insights, to support, strengthen, and rehabilitate broken people. Life consists of highs and lows, and rather than fear them, we can recognise that these difficult experiences are intrinsic to the human experience.

The Ghoul of S.A.D.

Kamilah McInnis-Neil

It flees the nest for wonders abroad
Because your sun is shining
It seeks a victim overseas
Like you, who's just surviving

Its presence receding, gradually leaving
A truce to your internal fight
It's packed its bags to blight new shores
And finally caught its flight

Goodbye! *Au revoir! Arrivederci* to the cretin!
That feeds upon your might
And though you revel in its welcome departure
A return is often in sight

The time has come for 'Hot Girl Summer'
The plan? To strut and flirt
With naughty innuendos, nights filled with crescendos
. . . though some will end in hurt

Pre-drinks, a party,
And don't forget afters,

The odd walk of shame?
Not the worst of disasters,
You walk, you talk,
You dance, you groove,
We sing, we shout,
We shake, *we move*

You close your eyes, the seasons change
Those feelings emerge, still lurking
You blast it with your lamp of light
The demon within still smirking

Its clutch this time is slippery
Although its visits recurring
The overwhelming days still come
But the tools you've learnt *are* working.

100 mg

Furaha Asani

Send tweet.

> *Today is #WorldMentalHealthDay and I'd like to share that a few days ago my GP and I decided that I need to double my dosage of sertraline from 50 mg to 100 mg daily. There is no shame in needing various support mechanisms, and adjusting/adapting them, to cope with mental illness.*
> 9:42 AM · Oct 10, 2021· Twitter for Android

Just under 280 characters to describe the end result of just over 280 weeks of my life, beginning in March 2016 when my father passed away unexpectedly. Though, if I'm being honest, the time-lines are blurry and bleed into each other. Anxiety clouds even my earliest memories.

9:42 AM · Oct 10, 2021

27 years away from obsessively scraping at my hands every time I washed them to get the dirt off;

25 years from silently pleading with God for forgiveness because I was scared I might have unknowingly sold my soul to the devil;

20 years from becoming convinced I had lost my ability to fall asleep;

14 years from when I had my worst crisis and feared I was losing my mind;

8 from the onset of intense hypochondria;

5 from the genesis of the grief I often fear will kill me;

2.5 from the border laws that nearly did kill me;

4 days from deciding with my doctor that it was the right time to double my dosage of sertraline from my daily 50 mg to 100 mg.

This drug will save my life.

For much of my early adulthood, internalised stigma and a misunderstanding of psychotropic drugs stopped me from seeking help via medication. Instead, I primarily relied on self-help mechanisms, holding myself together with invisible plasters and prayer.

Towards the end of his life, which coincided with when I embodied my ministry of mental health advocacy, my father became open about his own struggles with depression and his need for medication. Here was one of the firmest epitomes of strength in my life, demonstrating that he, too, needed a lifeline. A physician by profession, he was openly choosing to save himself by humbly asking for medication.

His unexpected death in 2016 marked the beginning of an intense period of grief and turbulence. His passing forced me to reckon with my own life: what would it take for me to want to live despite his absence, especially within a mind that was already teetering on the edge? The love of family and friends is a balm for a broken heart, but it doesn't always translate to a cure for illness.

Love is absolutely necessary for life, and I mean this not just in the physical sense but the psychological as well. The energy of love emanating from others has often resuscitated my deadened spirit. But love, even self-love, has not been enough to chase away the shadows that hide in the cobwebbed corners of my mind. Yet what love, and yes, self-love, too, has done for me is illuminate the roadmap for my healing. And this roadmap involves drugs.

From early 2017, I took 50 mg of sertraline daily, except for the days I forgot to. And the times I rationed my medication because I was running out of my prescription, because I no longer had access to the NHS, because I was fighting deportation from the UK, and my immigration status barred me from accessing free healthcare.

Looking back, I can see no way I would have been able to cope with my grief, anxiety and OCD over the past few years without this selective serotonin reuptake inhibitor (SSRI). One week into first taking it and the edge of my anxiety was taken off. It was no miracle cure, but it certainly was the ease that I needed at such a painful and unbearable time in my life.

Being cut off from the NHS resulted in me accepting 'donations' of sertraline from friends and friends-of-friends via the post. These donations kept me going for over one year. With my case now resolved, I'm registered with a new GP, and my prescriptions are back on course.

At the start of my journey on sertraline, I had the idea that I would likely need medication for a couple of years and then try to wean off them with support. I figured I'd be in therapy by then and ready to adjust my coping mechanisms. Life had other plans.

It isn't always easy to admit you are broken, especially when life's circumstances have pressured you into always having to display, and even perform, strength to get you through the day, or so your loved ones won't have another worry, or even so you don't let down those who are counting on your strength to catalyse theirs. There is relief, however, in letting go. There is freedom in divesting from the label of 'strong' and assessing your needs in the present moment. There is also an added layer of freedom in accepting that part of your personal evolution will encompass changing mental health needs and, therefore, adaptable coping strategies.

My journey with medication started with misinformed naivete. I now see that my assumption that I would need SSRIs 'only for a while' was deeply steeped in internalised stigma and maybe even ego – the expectation that my system 'should' eventually be able to wean off medication and cope on its own. I am now choosing to forgive myself for this false belief and intentionally rejecting this stigma.

I am not okay, but I am hopeful that I can find my way to a new version of 'okay'. And in just a few days of taking my double dose, I can feel the difference.

In this new phase of my experience with medication, I am also choosing not to place any timelines on my journey. Instead, my aim is to live as mentally well as I can, and I will incorporate a range of tools that help me meet my objectives. This includes beginning my day with 100 mg of sertraline. Shamelessly.

The Depression Cookbook

Rianna Walcott

At rock bottom

Hunger evades you for hours because you are conserving energy, laying very still, cocooned in your duvet, wondering if you can skip this whole day and try again tomorrow. You move at a glacial pace, make abortive attempts to roll out of bed, swaddled securely and helplessly as an infant awaiting liberation.

Surface.

Order (another) souvlaki. The deliveryman knows you by name, asks why you don't simply collect it from the restaurant that is just five minutes away. Burn with shame.

Head above water, gasping

Do you have a vegetable? Do you have a carb? Put the vegetable in a pan, stir-fry and always season. Gently weep as you mix it with the carb (probably pasta). Best accompanied with your four-day-old dressing gown and may be eaten directly from the pan with the silicone spoon you used to stir it with, if need be.

Mania

This time, you are sure your increased energy and desire to bake must be a good thing; you must be on the mend. Fill the home with guests, because baking is for company, and who knows when you'll feel this good again; this magnanimous; this urge to nurture yourself and others? Start out simple with banana bread muffins, cascade into crackled and crusty sourdough, personalised pizzas, flaky and golden patties, lemon drizzle cake, endless wheaten offerings that you pass around and guzzle down, and you see, I am well, you see how I can focus, could a depressed person do this?

When you surface again

you make a vat of chilli. Smile sagely as you mix in diced sautéed vegetables, let the smile turn smug as you sprinkle bay leaves, liberally add glugs of red wine, which is allowed, because you aren't drinking it directly. You've got this.

Violet

And sometimes, we see in violet. We see in dreams and visions, we see through fervour, we see the otherworldly.

Disclaimer.

Mica Montana

i do not mean to make psychosis
seem romantic
but neither will i accept
that the experience is tragic.

let's just say
it is part of what happens
when a universe discovers
it is wrapped in human fabric.

Self-Discovery

Mica Montana

when i tell you
that aliens have implanted
chips in my head
or that the CIA is leaving microphones
under my bed
that i
think i am Jesus,
don't get caught on the metaphors.

don't try to take my poetry
and fit it into your theory of psychology
In an attempt
to calculate how far away i am
from the normal way that a human being
relates to itself,
don't lock me into your definitions of mental health.
no, i don't actually think that i am Jesus of Nazareth
who walked the desert for forty days
and brought salvation through death.
what i am trying to communicate
is that i now recognize myself,
as important.

as having a cross to bear.
as a being made of love.
as a being, with a great purpose.
as a being, with a strong spirit.
so don't get upset
when i refuse to let you convince me
that it is irrational to feel like a God
when i have finally encountered
my divinity
when i have promised myself
to no longer let
the demons, the CIA, the aliens,
my negative thoughts
win in their attempt to
put out my fire.
win in their attempt to silence me
or turn me into something i don't want to be
so when i tell you
that i am fighting the aliens in my head,
that i'm getting rid of the microphones
that the CIA have put under my bed
that i
feel like Jesus.
don't get caught on the metaphors.
simply reply,
it's about time.

Disorderly Thoughts

Merrie Joy Williams

I remember shouting down a stairwell.
Wild and unhinged things would answer back.
Siblings crazed with the power of older children.
Ma's pot lids cymballing the pied kitchen walls,

half-green as closely guarded envy,
half-pink as a girl half-caught in gender's rusty chains.
The possibility of falling warned me,
hold on to the upstairs rails.

I recall jumping, unafraid flailing,
my feet aloft in quickened air.
Down fifteen jagged, jutting steps
it was a mighty arc – or death!

I'd land clean. On both feet.
No gymnast's extra step off beam,
the first thing in my life done well,
I lived for jumping after that.

I recall jumping
but were the jumps imagined? Real?

One thing which happened for certain, I feel,
Pa seemed far when needed close,

I did not see his bouts with ghosts, beyond
our door. The few that won were nothing to
the thousands more. And was his drink or
were my jumps the triggers of his violence?

And is it real or costume blood
deep in the downstairs carpet?
False memories, true memories,
both call from the bottom of stairwells.

The future, silent, behind them.

God Forbid

Tarek Younis

Ahmed pressed his hands against the armrests of his chair, but this brought him no relief. They continued their screaming.

'I'm not like you,' Ahmed told them. 'I seek refuge with God. May He throw you both in Hell.'

Ahmed watched his hands dance towards the space between his knees and form a broken vessel. His chest tightened: now they mocked his prayer, too. At least the waiting room was empty – thank God. He didn't want strangers thinking he was a beggar.

Indeed, Ahmed didn't want strangers seeing him here at all. He was supposed to be above this. Better than this. He had always thought of psychology as a deflection of the heart's spiritual diseases – a clever way to make excuses for amorality, really.

The waiting room was very small, its beige walls lined with six wooden armchairs, and a small table at its centre piled with magazines and mental health pamphlets. On top of the pile was this morning's newspaper, coffee-stained, with the headline: NINE TERROR PLOTS FOILED IN THE UK IN THE PAST YEAR, SECURITY SERVICES REVEAL. Ahmed suddenly felt acutely aware of his Muslim-ness. The newspaper wasn't entirely to blame for that – no, it was the room, its very air was not intended for people like him. Sitting here, trapped in one of its chairs, felt like a defeat, an indignity extending beyond himself to all of his kind.

At that moment, the large burgundy door leading to the therapy room opened, releasing an adolescent girl who walked past Ahmed, seemingly awash in a benevolent calm. Dr Brown appeared in the doorway, beckoning Ahmed with a nod. 'Alright,' thought Ahmed, 'we're doing this.' He interlocked his fingers close to his chest and went in.

Dr Brown's office was small, sparsely furnished with unremarkable things. A drippy coffee mug sat abandoned on a narrow desk, under a rectangular window with white blinds. A mustard-yellow couch awaited Ahmed on the far side of the room, where he took his seat. He felt silly: for some reason, he had expected a long chair.

Dr Brown sat down across from Ahmed, on a wingback chair covered in shiny, wine-red leather. It suddenly occurred to Ahmed the deliberate layout of Dr Brown's office: the doctor sat close to the door, a safe distance from his patients, ready to leave should they become erratic. *I am the patient*, thought Ahmed, and sank deeper into the couch.

Dr Brown was as Ahmed had expected: a middle-aged man with a face as round as a ball, blue eyes, a dingy nose and a receding hairline of short, brown hair. He wore Specsavers glasses and khakis with his shirt tucked in, a combination that didn't do his figure any favours. Dr Brown was white, but Ahmed also didn't expect water to be anything but wet.

Two large framed pictures hung side by side on the wall above Dr Brown's head. One was a photograph of a flower picture with a caption underneath it:

THE REAL YOU IS BURIED BENEATH THE SOIL. GIVE IT LIGHT – LET IT FLOURISH – BECOME THE REAL YOU.

The other square frame housed just two words:

JUDGEMENT-FREE ROOM.

Ahmed didn't care much for flowers or motivational bullshit, but the word *'judgement-free'* sat even more awkwardly with him. Judgement-free – what kind of fluff was that, exactly? He should have done more research before picking a therapist. He sorely wished for a Muslim, but all the specialists with Muslim names he'd found were female, and the only Muslim male had been booked for months. Ahmed knew he couldn't afford to wait, but he couldn't speak of *it* to a woman, either.

'Tacky, right?' Dr Brown smiled and pointed at the picture above his head. 'My wife told me I needed something to liven up the room. I can't say I agree. After all, we're not flowers – we are complex bio-psycho-social creatures. Anyway, I tell myself it's nice to look at. Good ice-breaker, too,' Dr Brown winked. 'Shall we get started?'

Ahmed's hands shuffled beneath him, and their twiddling movements made him self-conscious. He was a big guy, tall and bulky. No one ever pegged him as a twenty-two-year-old. For this meeting, Ahmed had ditched the ankle-length robe he normally wore on Fridays and dressed casually by design: blue jeans, Timberlands, a zip-up sports jacket with the collar popped. Ahmed didn't want to invite assumptions, though he still worried what Dr Brown would think of his beard – a fiery, wild, brown thicket. And there was no hiding his burning scalp, angry and inflamed from an aggressive shaving two nights ago. I must look crazy, thought Ahmed, and then remembered where he was.

Dr Brown explained the modalities of their relationship, his hands clasping and unclasping as he spoke, as if in self-applause. He listed the number of sessions available, the fee schedule, cancellation policies, and then, the confidentiality clause:

'Of course, everything you say remains between us,' said Dr Brown. 'I will never reveal anything identifiable to you outside of this room except in *extreme* circumstances – a point I tell all my patients. In situations of self-harm or harm to others, I may have to contact the police or a local authority. Do you understand?'

Ahmed acknowledged the exposition with a thoughtless nod but wondered: would harming one's soul count?

'I read your intake evaluation, Ahmed,' Dr Brown continued, flipping over loose papers in his hands as if to illustrate the point. 'You've reported experiencing anxious thoughts. You were having trouble falling asleep. You said you had lost your appetite.'

Ahmed met Dr Brown's questioning gaze and nodded in agreement: yes, yes, and yes. 'But that's not why you're here,' his hands sang in a children's tune, taunting him. 'Tell us, Ahmed, is there salvation in this room?'

Ahmed pressed the backs of his hands harder against his thighs. Their chanting turned to screams, which seemed to come from every bone in every finger, every muscle, every inch of skin. Wailing, crying, pleading. *Don't speak; don't tell him anything. Go home. We're sorry, we promise to be good. We'll listen to you. Let bygones be bygones. God will forgive you. God will forgive us. But you have to keep our secret. Don't you want to be forgiven?*

Ahmed's chest tightened and his heart pounded at his throat. There was no going back: strange boats had already crossed the hallowed ocean whose waters once shielded his secret, and now their hulls were about to touch shore and breach the sanctity of his deepest privacy. Ahmed drew a deep breath and let out a discreet '*bismillah*', disguising the blessed whisper by pretending to wet his lips.

'I'm . . . Uh . . . I have, um . . .' he stumbled. 'I have a problem with pornography.'

Ahmed's chest immediately tightened. He wished he could breathe back the words, but instead, felt suffocated. There was no turning back; the doctor's gaze had just breached the sanctity of his most private affair, and this door would forever remain open between them.

'I see this is quite distressful for you, Ahmed,' said Dr Brown gently, 'and I applaud your courage in coming here and opening up to me.'

Ahmed nodded. He felt a trace amount of light inside him, and it felt nourishing. Dr Brown was smiling as he continued:

'You know, Ahmed, there was once a group of researchers at the University of Montreal who conducted a study. The researchers needed participants who had never watched pornography before, and you know what?'

Dr Brown paused for effect, and delivered his punch line: 'They couldn't find any. Do you see where I'm going with this? You are certainly not alone and there is nothing to be ashamed of. I can see, however, that this habit is causing you distress. Perhaps you can elaborate on what is it about watching pornography that you find so upsetting?'

Ahmed could not prevent his head from jolting. The psychologist may as well have asked him to explain which part of a poison was lethal. Dr Brown's words of reassurance made it plain enough: he failed to see the problem. Ahmed realised that to answer Dr Brown's question, he'd have to start from the beginning – *the* beginning.

'Well, you see, Dr Brown, God created the heavens and the earth . . .'

Ahmed was prone to overthinking his issues, but this was his comfort zone, and so on he went: how Adam and Eve first recognised their nakedness, how men and women (especially men) were created with sexual drives that primed at the sight of nakedness, how sex is the primordial act of intimacy between husband and wife, how sex outside of marriage is an abomination towards God and society (especially God), how knowingly violating sacred prohibitions is a grave sin . . . Sweat gathered across his brow as he spoke. Ahmed was once told that, given the opportunity to explain Islam, he had better *perform*. Even as he ran out of words, Ahmed knew so much was left unsaid and wished he had been more articulate. There was so much at stake.

'In other words, you believe,' Dr Brown interrupted, 'that you have . . . upset God?'

'Yes,' said Ahmed. 'Yes, I have. Many times.' Ahmed doubled over, digging his elbows into his knees. His hands clenched at the non-existent hair on his clean-shaven, blistering scalp. Ahmed always shaved his head after lapsing, a ritual that was supposed to mark a new beginning. This time he was especially ferocious with the razor. The blade has long gone dull.

'When was the last time you saw pornography?' Dr Brown asked.

'Two nights ago.'

'Can you tell me what happened?'

Ahmed sighed and nodded. 'Okay, so, we have finals coming up. I study engineering, mechanical. I never wanted to get into engineering, but I did it for my dad. He's a mechanical engineer, too, you understand? I find it hard to study – really hard. To be honest, I hate it. My friends, my family, they see me sitting in front of books, they think I study a lot, that I'm a genius. But my relationship with books is . . . platonic, I guess? I don't care to look inside.'

Ahmed's cheeks began quivering uncontrollably and the struggle to retake control of his face produced an ugly grimace.

'I get . . . antsy, you know? When I need to study, I feel this tension, like something is burning inside me. It's always been there, even when I was a kid. Except then, it used to start in my chest, and now, it starts – it starts between my legs, and when it happens, I'm like a different person, I can't control myself, you understand? My hands . . . *my fucking hands.* They just do what they want to do, go where they want to go. One goes on the keyboard, and the other . . . you understand?'

Ahmed looked down at his hands. He'd been crushing them so hard between his knees they'd turned tomato-red. When Ahmed looked back at Dr Brown, he thought the man was eyeing his hands, too. He pushed them further down, out of sight.

'I'm sorry, Ahmed,' said Dr Brown, 'I can see this is very difficult for you.' Dr Brown looked at his papers, as if to spare Ahmed the shame of eye contact. 'So: you felt an agitation and masturbated?'

Ahmed quivered violently at the word. His face turned pale. He pushed himself to keep talking, to fill the awkward silence that seemed to quickly take the room.

'Two nights ago, I had to study for an exam – thermodynamics. I knew it would come – the urge – I knew I had to be ready. I needed a mental barrier, something to shut it out. So, I played the Qur'an off my phone. I turned it up really loud, and I sat down to study. Then, sure enough, there it was again. I delayed it, distracted myself, you know, Facebook, news videos, things like that, and the Qur'an was playing the whole time. I kept telling myself, 'How stupid would it be, doing *it* with the Qur'an in the background? It's the Qur'an, our Holy Book, you understand? What kind of idiot would even think about *it?* I'll tell you: someone fucked-up like me, apparently.'

Ahmed closed his eyes and drew a deep breath. It felt as if the air seared his pipes on its way in. He could feel his chest heaving erratically, could hear his voice turning shrill as he continued speaking, but his hands – they remained firmly locked between his knees. Ahmed was not going to let them go, so help him God.

'So, three hours later, I still haven't opened my book, and I knew it was over. I knew *it* won, I knew it. I wanted to get it over with, but I had to turn the Qur'an off, I couldn't just do it with the Qur'an there, you understand? I picked up the phone, but it froze – black screen. The Qur'an kept playing, I couldn't lower the volume, I hard-reset but even then it wouldn't stop! I live in a studio apartment, do you understand? I put the phone inside the fridge, but I could still hear it! I couldn't put it in the bathroom with the Qur'an playing, do you understand? I stuffed the phone deep inside my closet and piled all my clothes on top of it, but I could still hear it! I threw my blankets and pillows on top of the heap, pushed the closet door shut, then took my mattress and pushed it against the closet door. The sound became muffled, but I could still hear it! I put headphones in my ears, but I could still hear it, do you understand? Do you understand?'

Ahmed froze suddenly and collapsed sideways unto the couch. The intense anguish blooming inside him had grown denser and denser until it imploded, leaving behind a black hole that drained any light that remained in his chest. Ahmed's hands remained pinned between his knees by some mysterious force.

'I just had to wait for the battery to die, all I had to do was wait for the battery to die,' he whispered. 'I couldn't even do that. I did the thing that I did, but I could still hear it. I did the thing that I did, but I could still hear it.'

The crescendo was followed by six minutes of silence. Ahmed's body was stiff and still as a husk, and the odd, muted gasps emanating from his chest were its only signs of life. Dr Brown said nothing.

'Do you think God will forgive us?' Ahmed finally whispered. His lips barely moved as he spoke, like a ventriloquist; his voice seemed to emanate from somewhere on the periphery of his body.

Dr Brown stared at Ahmed with eyes wide open, either in concern or confusion. 'I can see this is very distressing for you – to fall out of grace with God,' Dr Brown said. 'Have you tried any . . . spiritual counselling? Consulted a Muslim priest?' Dr Brown asked.

'I did,' the husk of Ahmed replied. 'More than once. I tried everything.'

'And they couldn't help you?' asked Dr Brown.

'They told me I needed to stop, that I was burning my good deeds. Everyone reminded me not to despair, to be certain it will get better. I think my despair worsened with every reminder. The last imam I spoke to – his name is Sheikh Abdul-Azim – he told me that I needed help, that I can't do it on my own. He told me I should go see a psychologist. So, I came here.'

Dr Brown smiled, shuffled his legs and leaned back in his chair. 'I think I can help you,' he said, smiling. 'You see, I have experience treating addictions – and what you're struggling with is, at its core, an addiction.'

The husk that was left of Ahmed revived immediately at the encouraging words, grasping at the promise of help. He sat up.

'Well, I won't sugar-coat it,' Dr Brown replied to the sudden movement, 'addictions are difficult. But I see you're determined, and if you're willing to do what must be done, you'll overcome it.'

'But . . . you're going to help us stop, right?' Ahmed asked. 'You have to help us . . . Otherwise, how could God forgive us?'

Ahmed was whispering, but they were urgent whispers that made plain his desperation. Ahmed ignored the puzzled expression that settled on Dr Brown's face, and his reluctance to answer.

'What do you mean by *us*, Ahmed?' Dr Brown asked.

'Hmm?'

'Why do you ask if God will forgive *us*?'

Ahmed's face convulsed. He felt exposed and vulnerable. He hadn't realised what he was saying. His hands unshackled from their hold and ran free. The fingers twirled mockingly in the air, liberated.

'I . . . Uh, I meant *me*,' mumbled Ahmed. 'Sometimes when I'm out of it, you know, I . . . I talk about my body like it's . . . a different person, I guess? But it's just – it's nothing, it's just the way I talk sometimes. I'm not . . . I'm not here about *that*. Like you said, I have an addiction. That's why I'm here. Can we deal with that?'

Ahmed saw Dr Brown deflate in his seat, and this devastated him. The burgeoning tension emanating from his lower back now spread across his limbs like wildfire, and his body answered with a downpour of perspiration. It took all of Ahmed's willpower to stay seated; the edges of his body taunted him to run – now, and quickly.

Two minutes of infinite silence passed, until Dr Brown finally leaned forward and knotted his hands together, almost pleadingly.

'Ahmed, imagine, if you will, that your body *was* actually a different person. Imagine it sat with you on the couch right now. What would you say to it?'

Ahmed felt a chill. He didn't have to *imagine* – it was there immediately, sitting by his side on the couch, like a spirit summoned. It looked like Ahmed, dressed like Ahmed – but its smirk was not his. It smiled something else. Ahmed's heart fell like a stone to his abdomen. Only God knew of his relations with his body. Yet here it was now, Ahmed's divorced chassis: no longer concealed in the mind's eye, but sitting beside him as if in a family session.

Ahmed couldn't remember the moment the rupture first occurred, but on some level, he knew. It had been with him since childhood, or rather at the end of it, when so-and-so did such-and-such to him. He had no words to speak of it then, and it was all but forgotten now – translucent memories imprinted skin-deep, without subjects or objects or verbs. Ahmed would not let them in any deeper. It was no surprise that Ahmed was prone to addiction; anything that made him forget his *self*. Pornography was good for that, but when Ahmed found faith, at fifteen, the consumption began searing into his flesh.

'Yes, Ahmed, what would you say to me?' Ahmed's body repeated Dr Brown's question, smiling a devilish smile.

Ahmed turned towards his doppelganger, and his face turned crimson. He could not hide the malice he harboured towards it.

'I would tell it . . . I would tell *you* that I have nothing to do with you. You are damned and cursed, and you will not drag me to hell with you.'

'But don't you like it, Ahmed?' the sneering apparition replied. 'How it feels? *So* delectable. Besides, you are the one who commands *me*. Am I not your obedient servant?'

'I don't command you!' screamed Ahmed, too livid to worry about the startled Dr Brown jumping in his seat. 'I *never* told you to do these things. *You've* always done what *you've* wanted. Please God—' Ahmed's hands clasped his face, '—don't hold me accountable for the things my body has done.'

'But Ahmed, dear Ahmed . . .' The apparition tapped its chest at the spot where the heart should be. 'I'm empty inside. I'm just a shell. Will you tell God that I am to blame for your misery? Fine, go ahead. I will ask Him to judge the one who holds the heart! Remember? *"There's no man on earth born of two hearts".*'

Ahmed choked and tears streamed down his cheeks. He felt each breath explode in his chest, and his torso heaved fast, forcefully. This lasted a minute and then, all at once, Ahmed was still. A sudden and unfamiliar sensation overwhelmed him. What was it? It felt like *relief,* but it arrived so unexpectedly, Ahmed was unable to process it. He grabbed his head and dragged it between his legs, his hands and knees forming a cage around it.

'God, I just wish I can get away from this fucking body!' Ahmed sobbed from his prison. 'I'd do anything to get away! Anything – for you, oh God!'

Dr Brown sat silent, unmoving, his mouth slightly agape. At first, it was the intensity of Ahmed's anguish that had startled Dr Brown. Looking at the tense, red-faced, twisted man before him, Dr Brown was bracing for a murder confession – not a common porn addiction. Dr Brown was, of course, not oblivious to the anxious substructures underlying addictions, but this was different. This was depersonalisation. Dr Brown had only two previous clients who experienced such severe dissociation. Both had been white adolescent girls who suffered terrible abuse in childhood, and were coping with the trauma by distancing themselves from their wounded bodies. *Do devout Muslims actually experience trauma from masturbation?* thought Dr Brown. So many questions . . . but the day had been long and this patient, his body coiled around his burning scalp, had been exhausting.

When Ahmed began talking to his body, it was with such intensity, Dr Brown thought he heard the body speak back. Then, *it appeared.* Dr Brown could see *it* now, too. He jumped in terror and clung to his chair, resisting the urge to bolt out the door. Dr Brown retained enough composure to place two fingers on his jugular vein, and counted his pulse until ten. He quickly deliberated over every possible explanation for what his eyes couldn't stop seeing: *two Ahmeds* on his couch. The wretched soul and the cruel body by his side.

It must be stress, concluded Dr Brown, *an illusion born of stress. Ahmed's intense anguish projected into my visual cortex. It doesn't matter that I see it; it* belongs *to Ahmed.* He let out his breath. The thought reassured him enough, for the moment at least.

'I see this must be very difficult for you,' Dr Brown said, but his voice trailed off. The apparition was too vivid. *Who* was he addressing? Who was he *supposed* to address?

Ahmed did not respond anyway; neither did his double. As the coiled Ahmed cooed at its side, the apparition seemed to watch Dr Brown with great intent, as if anticipating a conversation.

Dr Brown fell silent once more. For the first time in twenty years, he felt like a man lost in his craft. Patients were often much simpler than this, but everything about Ahmed seemed strange and foreign, and Dr Brown was stifled by his disorientation. *The patient's culture has no bearing on the treatment*, he'd reminded himself again. *But this apparition . . .*

'It's true,' said a voice. Dr Brown recoiled in his chair, afraid the apparition could hear his thoughts, but it was the real Ahmed speaking. The man's head had emerged from the captivity of his limbs, seemingly out of sheer exhaustion. Ahmed looked strangely pleased, as if he'd gotten answers, though Dr Brown had yet to give any.

'What is?' responded Dr Brown, now deliberating on how to end the session as soon as possible.

'What it says, under that flower picture,' continued Ahmed. 'Maybe things *do* just need a little light sometimes. Someone told me once that there's a cure for everything in this world – except death. I think I've forgotten that.' Ahmed patted himself on the chest, a faint glimmer on his face. 'I feel lighter somehow, like I've had this boulder on my chest for a long time, you know? It was so difficult to breathe. But speaking with you today – I feel like it's nudged the boulder a bit. I didn't want to come here, not really, but I really *would* like to continue. It's an amazing feeling to be . . . *undamned*, you know?'

Dr Brown smiled reflexively, thanked Ahmed for coming, and stood up. Ahmed understood. The young man walked up to the door and extended his right hand towards Dr Brown's gut, where all the feelings churned in confusion.

'Same time next week, is it?'

Dr Brown nodded, shook Ahmed's hand with his right and

opened the door with his left. As soon as Ahmed walked out, Dr Brown shut the door and turned nervously towards the couch. His heart quivered: *Ahmed's double* was still there. What was it? *Whose* was it now?

'Pathetic, isn't he?' The apparition moulded its lips – Ahmed's lips – into a mischievous smile. 'You should have told him: there's no room for God in therapy, right?'

'What– what do you want?' Dr Brown asked shakily.

'Me? I don't want anything. I don't even know why Ahmed brought me here. He's already dragged me to every mosque in the city, to all those moralising imams, and what? No one's got a fix. What was he thinking – that you'll give him a magic pill and I'll go away? Or you'll teach him how to control me? He's always had that awful look with me, full of hatred. Like I'm the bad guy here!'

Dr Brown sank deeper into his seat. He was utterly baffled: was he really doing this? Was he actually having a session with an apparition? Dr Brown couldn't bring himself to speak. Meanwhile, Ahmed's double seemed to share his owner's propensity to monologue.

'Look, doctor, let's be honest here,' the apparition said with a ghastly chuckle. 'You really think you can help this guy? C'mon. I know him better than you – *I'm him.* You think he believes in this . . . this *psycho*-therapy? The spectre slapped his leg and pointed at Dr Brown. 'You! He doesn't even like you. He thinks you're full of shit!

'There's nothing you can do,' pressed the apparition. 'Ahmed doesn't want your help. *We* don't want your help. All Ahmed wants is heaven, can't you see? People like you, like those imams, all you give are promises, promises, promises . . . What if I found Ahmed a *guarantee*? There's more to the internet than girls, I've seen it. Hah! Let me show it to Ahmed, and see if he comes back to you. Oh, he's so *desperate*. And if I give Ahmed the *guarantee*, how could he keep hating me? If I promised him he didn't have to suffer anymore, didn't have to struggle for heaven, won't he love me for it?' The eyes of the thing glowed with a fiery glaze. 'He's going to listen to me, I tell you, because I'm not going anywhere! You hear me, doctor? How does that make *you* feel?!'

Then it was gone, as if it never was. Dr Brown felt a nerve ignite his gut, where all his thoughts and feelings churned. What did he just see? What did he just hear? He saw psychological vulnerabilities everyday, but he'd never seen ghosts. Why had it appeared with Ahmed?

Shaken, Dr Brown tried to make sense of his confusion. The apparition strangely reminded him of the anti-radicalisation training he'd received three weeks ago, though he couldn't recall the details. It was something about distressed Muslims – no, wait, it wasn't about Muslims at all. No, it was something about *psychological vulnerabilities.* 'Mental professionals having a role to play in preventing terrorism,' he was told. 'It's *not* about Muslims.'

I'm the mental health professional, Dr Brown reminded himself. The thought provided little reassurance. In fact, it *terrified* him. He saw psychologically vulnerable individuals every day. None had come with an apparition.

Dr Brown rolled his chair to his desk to write his notes. He wrote with trepidation, weighing every word. The world might read them one day, he thought, in the event of – what? All this talk of God, hell, heaven, *guarantees*; which words had been Ahmed's, and which ones spat by the double? Dr Brown's thoughts were jumbled; the possibilities scared him even more.

Dr Brown wrote page after page, filled them with citations, observations, and personal thoughts, accounting for every minute of the fifty-minute hour he'd spent with Ahmed. The more he wrote, the less anxious he felt. If the apparition was an extension of Ahmed, a projection of his psyche, then it wasn't Dr Brown's problem at all. It was Ahmed's. *It was Ahmed.*

Dr Brown ensured his office would be *known* to function as a pre-criminal space, as he'd been instructed to. The first line of his final paragraph on the third page began, 'Ahmed presented potentially significant psychological vulnerability towards radicalisation,' and ended with, 'It will be important to keep a keen eye on Ahmed's development.'

Now, no one could point the finger at Dr Brown. He felt tremendous relief at this thought, like a boulder off his chest. Not that anything *should* happen, of course. No, but just in case . . .

The memory of the apparition flashed before Dr Brown, to which his gut responded with another churn. Dr Brown sighed and reached for his phone. He needed to tell someone about Ahmed. One can never be too cautious these days. Just in case – God forbid.

In Conversation with
the Editors

This interview was edited from a conversation that took place on 29 November 2021, shortly before the editors submitted the manuscript for this edition.

Samara Linton: A lot has happened in our lives since the first edition was published. For example, when we first started, you were at the beginning of your Ph.D, and now you're coming towards the end. Is that reflected in the book at all?

Rianna Walcott: Well, in 2018, when the book was first published, I was twenty-four, and now I'm a big woman, you know! I'm twenty-seven and have had so many more life experiences. When we first started this book, I had not had that much experience with therapy, had only just about started antidepressants; I was starting a new chapter of my life, and now I'm closing it up. It is not ideal that I've produced the same book twice during my Ph.D and neither of them are the book that I was supposed to produce, the actual thesis, but here we are.

I definitely feel like a totally different person from who I was at the beginning. Then, I was a person who was talking about mental health as a service user, as someone just getting to grips with it, as someone who was creating a resource because nothing like it existed, and I needed it. Whereas, now, a few years on, I'm someone who considers themselves an advocate. I'm someone who has worked with loads of different mental health organisations. I've got a little bit more confidence in what I'm talking about, in being able to be a helpful and useful force. And, I guess, just older, wiser, more jaded, but also more effective.

SL: Yeah, I feel that. When the book was first published, I had just started my first year as a doctor. I was literally working on an acute psychiatric ward. Fast-forward to now, I am no longer working as a doctor, I've made a huge career change, and I'm working in media, specifically radio and podcasting. I've gone through a huge transitional period. In fact, shortly after the book was published, my mental health reached the lowest that it ever has, and I had my own experiences of using secondary mental health services and hospitalisation and so on. So, I have been making these huge life changes and addressing some parts of my life that cause distress. So, I feel like I am editing this book with a sense of survival, having been through some of my lowest lows.

RW: 100 per cent.

SL: And then coming out the other side of that. I suppose it adds more gravity to the importance of this work, and I think I hold it with more reverence now. Like I need this book even more now than when I first started. I'm so grateful that I could turn to the experiences shared in this book while going through these really low lows because they made it a much less alienating experience. So, my work has always been shaped by my academic background and work in mental health and medicine, and I think now, the personal has become even more significant.

RW: This is one of those situations where having that lived experience makes you more of an authority. Maybe we wouldn't be the right people to have created this book otherwise. Maybe without those experiences, we wouldn't have been as sensitive, or have taken the care that we have with our contributors, especially with everything that happened with our last publisher, and wanting to really protect our contributors' safety and their ability to speak.

I think that part of what we've experienced in our own lives, with our own mental health, means we're able to treat people how we wanted to have been treated, and we're able to create the resource that we needed, and I think that that has been the biggest part of shaping this book.

SL: Yeah, exactly. Linked to that, beyond our own personal experiences of mental distress, has anything else shaped how we've approached this edition? Maybe more so for you, because of your Ph.D research?

RW: Well, I'm thinking about what happened with our previous publisher and the particularly digital, technological shitstorm that surrounded it, simultaneously making the trauma highly visible, and also providing a solution and support in that visibility. The whole point of this book is a response to white supremacy, a response to the trauma of working in – and suffering inside – predominantly white institutions in the UK. And then our very worst fears were confirmed, and it happened in such a public, such a callous, cold and digital way.

My research is on social media and online communities, the types of care and bonds we create in those spaces. And this work around communities of care, and Black feminism online in particular, really made it possible for us to bounce back from the experience. We would not have been able to shape this edition again without the support of various people in the digital space, people who were touched by our story and wanted to support us. People who wanted to help us and offered us free advice, looked over contracts, and put us in touch with the right people. People who retweeted, made our plight public, people who interviewed us and made sure our story got to the right places. We would never have been able to reclaim this narrative and reclaim this moment without them. It would have ended very badly and very sadly.

And even just with the format of this *In Conversation* being at the back of this book, that to me is a nod to some of the wonderful Black feminist texts that have shaped my work, and wanting to be part of this tradition of allowing for knowledge curation and discourse to happen in ways that are not just the traditional pen to paper. It's about being able to have a conversation, being able to have a dialogue, and then being able to print it in this way. Thinking about forms of knowledge production that aren't traditional has been especially helpful to me in my work throughout this Ph.D and throughout creating this edition. You know, thinking about the ways that my neurodivergence, in particular, helps and hinders my work; the fact that sometimes it's easier for me to dictate and have a conversation with someone than it is to write.

Also, thinking about neurodivergence and accessibility has been really embedded in this book. I mean, I'd say it was in our first edition too, you know, making sure that people were able to contribute in every way they could and wanted to. But I think we've just taken that to its logical conclusion here and really done more in terms of making sure that this work is accessible.

SL: Absolutely. And how has the editing process been this time around?

RW: I think one of the things that's been really great for me this time round is acknowledging how well you and I work together and thinking about where our strengths are. The fact that we're even able to get this done is a testament that you are wonderful at some things, and I can just about balance it out with the other sides.

SL: You're being incredibly modest! But I would agree that we know ourselves so much better this time around, and it's made the process so much more straightforward – simple things like division of labour.

RW: Having a good publisher . . .

SL: That too! It's a vastly different experience; they almost don't feel comparable. Having the wider support of an actual publishing team and agent, you know, relinquishing some of the responsibility, has been great.

RW: Yeah. I'm thinking about how you and I were so scarred and traumatised by the amount of labour we had to do the first time round, that when it came to something as simple as creating an index, we'd already started fretting about budgeting, about how we would do it ourselves or afford to pay someone to do it. And then we went, oh, maybe that's something we could ask the publisher, and they said, 'Oh yeah, obviously, we'll do that.' Come on, that's trauma!

SL: I think it's so telling. We had come to accept this feeling of being burdened by work as normal. Silently doing this labour is expected, right?

RW: It's instinctive for us to try and do it all ourselves.

SL: Absolutely, and I think that's something that you can see in a lot of the experiences in the book as well. It is so normal for us to labour, to suffer, to carry burdens. And then people realise that maybe it doesn't have to be that way; maybe there are ways that, as communities and as networks, we can alleviate that burden.

They realise the liberation that comes from that, and I think, in a way, our experience just illustrates that.

RW: Definitely. I certainly find it very difficult to ask for help. At the time of this conversation, I'm deep in the write-up for my Ph.D, and it has been a struggle. Yet, the thought of even asking for more time, the thought of asking you to help me out and pick up some of the slack on editing – it took me weeks to even muster the courage to ask for help, and this is with my own book about mental health. Like what is that?

SL: But I think we also need to give ourselves grace. Like we are young, we were younger the first time round, but we're still young now. And like everyone, we are still learning and growing, and this is part of that process. Compared to three years ago, we are doing absolutely brilliantly.

RW: Now, when we hit thirty, come on!

SL: Exactly! And, Rianna, you contributed your own piece this time around, 'The Depression Cookbook'. Tell me about that.

RW: So, I've been thinking a lot about neurodivergence and how certain things in my life play out as a result of that. I have a very complicated relationship with food, and certain traumas in my family, and 'The Depression Cookbook' is something I wrote in the midst of mania. I wrote it all on my iPhone notes in one sitting. Some months later, I came back to it, thinking about putting it in the book, and I realised that it was already done.

One of the poems that I really enjoy in the book is 'To Braise the Belly Right' by Minying Huang. It really resonated with me because she is the meal that is being cooked, and it got me thinking about depression in those terms and made me really reflect on my own practices of how I cook and when I cook.

Cooking is one of those markers that tells me how well I am. When you're in the midst of a depressive episode, for example, you just don't have the perspective or the distance to really understand what you're going through. It's all just very all-consuming. So, things like getting hyper-fixated on certain tasks, procrastinating by baking loads of food or putting up shelves, and putting all of your emotions into something that maybe to an outsider doesn't look very important, but then it goes wrong, and you're suddenly sobbing on the floor. So, sort of understanding how I externalise some of what goes on in my head was really cathartic because it helps me recognise those markers and track how I'm actually doing when it's not immediately clear to me.

SL: That makes a lot of sense.

RW: Why didn't you write a piece?

SL: I thought about it. It's not that I haven't got anything to write about; I definitely do. As I mentioned, you know the last three years have been so tumultuous; they've been such a period of change and transition. I think for me, I just decided that it wasn't the right time. The way my depression and anxiety manifests is, I am always terrified of letting opportunities pass me by.

RW: Oh my god, same.

SL: Yeah, I am always scared that if I don't take advantage of opportunity, it may never come again. Then, I would have let myself down, let everyone down; I'm going to regret this for the rest of my life blah blah blah, that spiral of thoughts. And I've been working really, really hard at challenging those assumptions and challenging the need to always produce and always be productive. I'm sure so many perfectionists can relate to that feeling of needing to produce something wonderful and brilliant, and if you don't, it really eats away at your core. And as someone who has grown up as a high achiever, leaving medicine without actually having a career plan or goal in mind was the beginning of this process of me saying that I don't need to grab hold of everything now. I don't need to take advantage of everything that passes me by. If it passes me by, and it never comes again, then so be it. So, coming back to why I didn't contribute my own piece, I just feel like it's not the time for me.

And you know, mental health is such a private and individual experience, but it is also relational and shared. My story is so intertwined with my family and my loved ones, the people I work with, and so on. The story that I want to tell is so much bigger than what I have the capacity to produce right now, and I just have to trust that one day I'll have the opportunity to really tell that story. And at the end of the day, I love editing. I love putting other people's work out there, and by not sharing my story right now, I have been able to dedicate more time and energy to that.

RW: I think that reasoning is absolutely wonderful, because I think there's so much to be said and so much for us to learn about resting. One of the ways that I've started to think about it is – if I don't write something new, if I don't create something new, do I stop being a writer? How many things do I have to make before I'm allowed to call myself one? I'm working on understanding that taking a rest and taking a break is better for us than continually pouring from an empty cup. One of the things that I'm looking forward to – and terrified of – is taking what I will call my 'fallow year', inspired by Theophina Gabriel's *Onyx* Magazine. Some time after my Ph.D, to rest, recover – and just really think about: what do I really want to do next? You know, not just constantly chugging forward and producing out of exhaustion.

SL: But it's terrifying, isn't it?

RW: It's so scary. Absolutely terrifying. There's obviously demands of life, like paying rent.

SL: And there's this real kind of identity challenge that you have to come to terms with.

RW: Oh my god, like, who will I be?

SL: Yeah, exactly.

RW: I wonder how that will be for my mental health; what happens when I am a person resting as opposed to someone who's getting their Ph.D and writing a book, etc.? How will I think of myself? How will I be thought of? I don't know. I'm very excited for it, and I'm also dreading it, and I think I'm definitely going to take inspiration from your reasoning to not write for this edition.

SL: I think we also need to remember: you and I are blessed with good networks and good communities and people who love us and people who will hold us.

RW: Absolutely. Why do we behave as though we don't have support? What do you hope that people will take away from this book?

SL: I hope they will take away . . . solidarity is such an over-used word, but I think it's this feeling of connectedness. The feeling that we are connected to so many experiences and lives and stories beyond our own, and it doesn't necessarily make your experience easier or better, but I think it kind of grounds it in something real and something kind of lasting. That gives me a lot of comfort, and I'm hoping it gives other people comfort too.

RW: I think comfort is a wonderful one. But I'm also hoping that we're on the cusp of a revolution.

SL: I love it.

RW: You know – enough is enough. Not enough has changed for the better since we published this book the first time around. I think the pandemic has thrown into sharp relief how disproportionately impacted communities of colour are across the UK and globally. You know, as we speak, the news media are starting to refer to the newest variant of Covid-19 as the 'South Africa variant', having learned nothing from calling it the 'China virus', you know? We are constantly made scapegoats, constantly made villains, and I think a lot of the discussions we've been exposed to over the pandemic about vaccine hesitancy in communities of colour are part of that process of us constantly being vilified for issues that are structural in nature. Something has to give, and something has to give quickly, so, I'm hoping for a revolution.

SL: I mean, if we have a community that is connected and rested, and you know, secure in themselves and their identity, how can we not have a revolution?

RW: Right? Bun Babylon.

Acknowledgements

To all our continuing contributors, thank you for entrusting us with your experiences, stories, and emotions for a second time. Thank you for your understanding, patience, and compassion during what turned out to be a turbulent journey. You are the rock upon which this book stands. To all our new contributors, thank you for choosing to be a part of this story. Thank you for sharing your lives with us and, in turn, giving this book new life.

Thank you to our agents Sophie Scard and Kat Aitken, to Bluebird for their support and for making this revised edition a reality.

We are grateful to Sharp Rights, who looked over our contract, making the return of the rights from the first edition a possibility. Thank you to the Society of Authors and Publishing Scotland for your invaluable advice, and to Professor Sunny Singh for her fierce championing of us when the bad news broke. To Mairi Oliver of Lighthouse Books, no words will ever be enough for the kindness and generosity you showed us. Thank you to everyone who reached out with love and support at every step of this journey – we could not have done this without you.

Samara

To Lucy and Robin for opening up your home and hearts to me, for providing a refuge in a world that can feel overwhelming. Thank you to India for making sense of my rambling voice notes. Tom and Mugabi, thank you for your guidance.

To everyone who pulled me out of the darkness that threatened to swallow me whole, you know who you are. The A & E staff, my home treatment team, Dr Sani, Dr Mehnaz. I am grateful to my colleagues on Ruby ward who treated me like family, to those patients who brought light to the bleakest of days. Thank you, Dami, for helping me laugh again. To Sandra, my ever-patient therapist. Thank you for giving me the tools to stand on my own two feet. To my loved ones, who gave me a reason to do so.

I am ever grateful to my wonderful friends: Nikki, Lwazi, Tiggy, Wandy, Tobi, Naomi, Ella & Ella, Rhianna, Robyn, Precious, Mike, Jackson, Ada, Tanya, Lolly, and Fausta. My fabulous neighbours: Darryl and Shadi. Rianna, my wonderful writing partner and confidante, may your light ever shine bright. Thank you to my dearest Rue.

I am grateful to my family, especially Aunty Marie and Aunty G, thank you for helping me feel less alone. Thank you, Grandma and Grandpa, my constant sources of love and encouragement. To my parents, Fitz and Rosie, thank you for helping me become the woman I am today, for holding me close even when it hurts. Thank you to my sister Anna, the most perfect gift God ever gave, to Robert and Sarai, my beating heart.

Rianna

I have a lot of thanks to give, because all my strength comes from the people I love, and who love me in return. To my colleagues, supervisors, mentors – in particular Dr Anouk Lang, Dr Zeena Feldman, and Dr Francesca Sobande. You all inspire me to be my best self, believe in me when I am unable to, and all that I am and have achieved I owe to you. To my therapist, Gloria, who is patiently teaching me how to have it all. Samara, thank you for tolerating me for yet another book, and for dragging us to the finish line. There is no better partner than you.

Thank you to Maïa – the better Walcott sibling, my soulmate, my favourite person on God's green earth. Thank you to Paris, my sister from before my sister came along. I am so grateful for the support and unconditional love of my parents, the overwhelming love of our matriarch, my grandma, and my grumpy old grandad who is completely incapable of hiding how much he adores us all.

To Olivia, Xine, 3ianna, Chloé, Maeve, Mim, Rick, Jackson, Lindsey, and countless others, it is my greatest privilege to call you all my friends.

To the Genderqueer Special Crimes Unit, my Queer Council: Jessica Brough, Jade Bentil, and Paula Akpan. You mean more to me than I can contain here but I will try: just being in community with you is a balm, an honour. You clear my vision and allow me to believe in the possibility of a better world.

About the Contributors

A. K. Niemogha (she/her) is a young Black Brit, passionate about making a difference in her community and social justice for all. A social worker within mental health services, she is learning to overcome writer's block.

Ailsa Fineron (she/her and they/them) is a trainee psychotherapeutic counsellor who also loves being creative in multiple media. Hailing from East Lothian, Scotland, they've lived in Bristol for the past decade.

Aimen Rafique-Marsh (she/her) lives and works in London, with her husband, Michael, and six-year-old tuxedo cat, Mars. Rafique-Marsh is a multidisciplinary visual and sound artist, and a published author. Her book, *Essays on Loss,* is available globally, via Apple Books.

Andrés N. Ordorica (he/him) is a queer, Latinx writer based in Edinburgh. He is a recipient of the Edwin Morgan Trust's Second Life grant. In 2021, he was shortlisted for both the Morley Prize for Unpublished Writers of Colour and the Mo Siewcharran Prize. He is the author of *At Least This I Know* (404 Ink).

Avila Diana Chidume (she/her) is an entrepreneur with a passion for art, diversity, and inclusion. In 2018, Avila founded Avila.Diana; a platform selling diverse greetings cards and gifts designed by artists from historically marginalised communities.

Becky Balfourth (she/her) is a 30-something-odd writer from east London. Spurred to write by the experience of mental illness and a general desire to express, she has had work published in *Mslexia* and on *Litro Online*, among other spaces. Her blog (about scars and recoveries) can be found at www.thesleevelessproject.com.

Caroline (she/her) is a young professional and mental health advocate based in Birmingham, passionate about raising awareness of mental health in the community.

Dr Cassie Addai (she/her) is Ghanaian-British, living in Scotland and working as a clinical psychologist, having completed her doctorate in 2019. Her doctoral thesis explored young people's experiences of refugee family reunion. Through her work, she hopes to empower people experiencing distress with a better understanding of their difficulties and ways of coping.

Cece Alexandra (she/they/them) is a Black, queer, non-binary woman. She has epilepsy, which she believes allows her to see the world through an intersectional and holistic lens. She is a passionate advocate for Black mental health and wellbeing. She is currently training to become an integrative counsellor and psychotherapist, and her goal is to work within the Black and LGBTQIA+ communities once she qualifies. Her creative and biographical writing on her personal mental health experiences has been featured on *HuffPost*, *The Mighty*, *Black Ballad*, and in the *Aspects of Faith* and *The Colour of Madness* anthologies. In her spare time she is a plant mother and music lover.

Christina Fonthes (she/her) is a Congolese-British writer. Her work, laden with themes of womanhood, religion and sexuality, has been widely published in journals and anthologies worldwide. Christina is the founder of REWRITE, a creative writing organisation for Black Women and women of colour writers around the globe. She is the winner of the Sky Arts Royal Society of Literature Writers Award for Fiction 2021. Christina lives in London. She is represented by Rocking Chair Books.

Corinne Crosbourne aka 'thewomanistwords' (she/her) is a Black-British woman of Jamaican heritage. After a gap year in South Africa, and while starting an undergraduate law degree, Corinne experienced a severe deviation from reality, but has learned to live with her mental health conditions since. She now works as an equality and diversity officer, studies Gender, Policy and Inequalities at London School of Economics, and is also a fine artist and poet.

Cynthia Oji (she/her) is a project manager living in east London whose keen interest in travelling and photography is depicted in her photograph 'LOVE', taken while in Rio De Janeiro, Brazil.

Dania Quadri (she/her) is a writer and medical student based in London. She has bylines in *gal-dem*, *burnt roti*, and *Roar Zine*. Say hi to her on Twitter @daniaq16

Danielle DZA Osajivbe-Williams (she/her and they/them) is an integrative counsellor and psychotherapist (MBACP), consultant, wellness practitioner, tarot diviner, Isese/Ifa practitioner, performance artist, lover of trees, and daughter of wisdom and freshwater. She plants seeds for liberation via wellness technologies of past/present/future.

David Sohanpal (he/him) is an asylum seeker who has fled persecution for speaking about the injustice back home and suffers from anxiety, depression and PTSD. Like many asylum seekers, he is not allowed to study or work while waiting for his status, which leaves many in a precarious situation, wasting their mind and rotting away.

Diljeet Kaur Bhachu (she/her) is a researcher, educator, musician, and activist based in Glasgow, Scotland. She has been writing poetry in various forms throughout her life but has only recently made it part of her main creative practice as a musician. Diljeet frequently collaborates with poets and spoken-word artists, setting their words to her music. You can hear and watch some of these collaborations at www.diljeetbhachu.com

Dylan Thind (he/him) is a computer programmer currently living in London.

Eljae's (she/her) writing has typically centred on the doing of relationships and how we construct ourselves as people. More recently she has been exploring Blackness, rest, and resistance, and feels privileged to once again be included in the necessary work of *The Colour of Madness*. Alongside accepting poetry commissions, Eljae is looking to develop her creative practice by exploring different mediums.

Esme Allman (she/her) is a poet, writer, theatre-maker, and facilitator based in south-east London. She works in a multi-disciplinary way exploring Blackness, desire, imagination, and the intersection of these themes. Esme has been commissioned by the Barbican Centre, BBC Radio 3, BBC Radio 6 and English Heritage. Her published work can be found in the Roundhouse Poetry Collective Anthology *We Have Never Seen Something Like This*, POSTSCRIPT, Barbican Young Poets' Anthology 19/20, and *The Skinny*.

Esther Kissiedu (she/her) is a British-born Ghanaian who uses storytelling to show different facets of the Ghanaian heritage and culture. She is an avid traveller and believes storytelling is a beautiful way to connect people to different cultural issues. At church, she works in the multimedia department to enhance the worship experience. And as Senior Digital Manager for Project Everyone, she works to promote the UN Global Goals.

Fahmida Liza Khan (she/her) is currently finishing off her Ph.D in Chemistry at the BP Institute via Shell Technology to focus on coatings for offshore energy structures at the University of Cambridge. She is also working as the Scientific Lead initially for the Covid-19 pandemic, but now expanding to DNA sequencing platforms and bioinformatics. Using her experience in energy landscapes and life sciences, she has joined corresponding organisations where she researches emerging technologies, sourcing scale-up investors for carbon-zero research in EMEA regions as well as being part of a team to build the Bangladesh Innovation Forum branch to source funding and develop early-stage biotechnology/climate-crisis ventures that will give back to society.

Farrah Riley Gray (she/her and they/them) is a Black Artist from south London, and graduated from Goldsmiths University in 2019. Their practice has a focus on misogynoir and the experiences of Black Women. Working through textiles, audio and text, they show how marginalised communities can be given representation within art and art spaces. Riley Gray was diagnosed with borderline personality disorder (BPD) in their mid-twenties.

Furaha Asani (she/her) is a public academic, mental health advocate, precarious migrant, and writer with interest in the themes of global health equity, a world without borders, and science in pop culture. She has written for several platforms including *Back Ballad*, *The Guardian*, *The Independent*, Forbes.com, *Medium*, *Star Trek*, *Huffpost*, and many others. Furaha loves pineapple ornaments and bold red lipstick.

Gold Maria Akanbi (she/her and they/them) is a bisexual, neurodiverse, British-Nigerian artist that works and studies in Liverpool and Oxford. Focusing on topics such as sexual feminism, the decolonisation of The Black (disabled) Body, epigenetic trauma and healing modalities and decolonised alternative spirituality, their performance work uses a range of formats to speak and interact with their audience, such as dance, gesture, silent film, sounds, poetry, and written text that accompanies said performance.

Haania Amir Waheed (she/her) is a lawyer by day and poet-cum-photographer in her free time. She has degrees in Creative Writing and Literature and Law. Moonlighting as a writer, Haania's work attempts to express the nuances of being a Pakistani Muslim caught between her birth and naturalised identities in the hope that someone, somewhere, finds it meaningful.

Hana Riaz (she/her) is a fiction writer and researcher who lives and loves in London. She is inspired by wholehearted communities and justice-led approaches to cities, living, and loving. Her short stories have been published by *The Good Journal*, Loss Lit, Peepal Tree Press, and the *As/Us* Journal. In 2019, she was longlisted for the London Short Story Prize.

Hima Chauhan (she/her) is a South Asian artist from Leicester. As a second-generation Gujarati immigrant, her art focuses primarily on the South Asian diaspora.

indyah (she/her and they/them) is a chronic overthinker and daydreamer; riding the waves of a mood disorder and self-soothing through scribblings.

Jason Paul Grant (Jason) is a lived experience consultant who uses knowledge, skills and experience to improve outcomes for people within the mental health system. Jason is currently working for Sussex Partnership NHS Foundation Trust, the Royal College of Psychiatrists, and the University of Manchester, working on a study looking into the ethnic inequalities in severe mental illness. Jason sits on various mental health advisory boards including the National

Institute for Health Research, Applied Research Collaborative for Kent, Surrey and Sussex; University College London's Institute of Mental Health; The Stability Network; and the Lived Experience Council for the Healthy Brains Global Initiative. Jason has degrees from Goldsmiths, University of London, City University London, University of Glasgow, and the Pathways to Success programme at the University of Oxford.

Javie Huxley (she/her) is a British-Chilean illustrator based in London, and the co-chair for the Save Latin Village campaign. Following Javie's MA in Children's Literature and Illustration, her main focus has been on socially engaged editorial illustration for magazines such as *gal-dem* and *Shado*. Javie strongly believes in the importance of art as advocacy, and her work focuses on themes such as identity and current social issues. Javie also uses her art to celebrate and platform Latinx voices in the UK. Find more of her work at @javhux and www.javiehuxley.com.

Jess Brough (they/them) is a writer, producer, and psycholinguistics Ph.D student at the University of Edinburgh. Jess is the founder of Fringe of Colour – an Edinburgh-based multi-award-winning arts initiative for Black people and people of colour. Their fiction can be found in *Extra Teeth, The Best of British Fantasy 2019* anthology and seed head, an anthology of new writing from The Future is Back series led by Olumide Popoola. Their non-fiction can be found at *gal-dem, The Skinny, The Bi-Bible: New Testimonials, Fringe of Colour*, and the Glasgow Film Festival.

Kalwinder Singh Dhindsa (he/him) is a Derby-born author, teacher and heritage enthusiast.

Kamal Kainth (she/her) is a Counselling Psychologist and Integrative Psychotherapist, who has worked in NHS mental health services for the past twenty years. She believes that therapeutic interventions should be systemic and dialogical, thereby encouraging individuals to construct their own narrative of their experiences. Kamal's writing is an attempt to begin conversations and to offer her reflections as a therapist, as a carer and as a client.

Kamilah McInnis-Neil (she/her) is a multimedia journalist at BBC News. She is extremely passionate about mental health. Having battled with depression, on and off for the past ten years, she uses art such as her music, journalism and poetry to express herself, turning pain into power. She is also a regular host and curator for Kind Fest, a digital festival that takes place on World Kindness Day, celebrating all things kind, while raising money for charities. When she isn't working, you'll find Kamilah playing the piano and violin, roller-skating or boogying at a festival.

Louisa Adjoa Parker (she/her) is a writer and poet of English-Ghanaian heritage who lives in south-west England. Her first poetry collections were published by Cinnamon Press, and her third, *How to Wear a Skin*, was published by Indigo Dreams. Her debut short-story collection, *Stay with Me*, was published in 2020 by Colenso Books. Her poetry pamphlet, *She Can Still Sing*, was published by Flipped Eye in June 2021, and she has a coastal memoir forthcoming with Little Toller Books.

Maïa Walcott (she/her) is a twenty-two-year-old Social Anthropology graduate from the University of Edinburgh. She is a multidisciplinary artist working with sculpture, painting, illustration, and photography. Her works have been exhibited widely, from publication of paintings on the Wellcome Collection's website, multiple illustrations with Project Myopia, an exhibition of her photography at Jupiter Artland and being hired as a photographer for vibrant photo exhibitions such as the I'm Tired Project and Celestial Bodies.

Merrie Joy Williams (she/her) is a poet, fiction writer, essayist, and writing tutor. She has won the Poetry Archive Wordview 2020 Competition, and been shortlisted or longlisted for the Bridport Prize, and the National Poetry Competition. Her debut collection, *Open Windows* (2019), is published by Waterloo Press.

Mica Montana (she/her) is an assistant research psychologist, mindfulness coach, workshop facilitator, mental health speaker, and poet. She holds degrees in Psychology, Philosophy and Neuroscience and in 2019 released her debut poetry collection *When Daisies Talk*, which explores her own personal experiences of psychosis. Since publishing, she has gone on to deliver art- and poetry-based mental health workshops across the UK and has spoken at various conferences, as well as appeared as a guest lecturer at the University of Leicester.

Michele D'Acosta (she/her) has a career spanning three decades across multiple art forms including filmmaking, creative writing, animation, painting, and digital art. Her sole purpose is 'to create positive social change'. Most recently, Michele was recognised as one of the sixty most influential BAME people in British Television by The TV Collective. Michele is best known as the producer of the critically acclaimed documentary film *Biggie & Tupac*, which has been named as one of the fifty most important documentary films from the past twenty-five years. Currently working on a memoir about her life as a Black adoptee raised by white parents in the conservative British countryside, Michele shines her lens deeply into the nuances of intersectionality, and how true healing can be achieved individually, locally, and globally.

Minying Huang (they/them) is an Oxford-based poet and writer. Their work appears in wildness, Palette Poetry, Electric Literature, and elsewhere. They are a Ph.D student in Medieval and Modern Languages and a Barbican Young Poet.

Miz Penner-Hashimoto (she/her and they/them) is a British Japanese playwright and multi-disciplinary artist based in New York City. Follow her on Twitter @mizbung

Neneh Patel (she/her) studied Illustration at Leeds Arts University and currently works in education. Her work focuses on the editorial, distilling an article or concept into a single image. Valuing the opportunity to work free-hand, Neneh enjoys playing with materials, and is drawn to flowing mediums, such as ink and watercolour. She chooses to work on a small scale during the developmental stages of her creative process and has also experimented with textiles and hand-sewing to translate sketched images into embroidered tapestry.

Niki M. Igbaroola (she/her) is Talent and Audience Development Manager at Cassava Republic Press where she champions literature from across the Black world. She is a writer and prolific reader, and a 2020 winner of the Stream Lyric Writers on Democracy commission. Niki has delivered workshops and chaired conversations at Africa Writes Festival and Aké Festival respectively, and continues to produce work to be delivered across different mediums.

Nisha Damji (they/them) is a queer, non-binary writer and organiser of South Asian descent. Nisha's areas of interest include mental health, migration and state violence. They live with ADHD, PTSD, and their little black cat, Rambo.

Ololade A. (she/her) was born and bred in London, England. By day, she works in the life sciences industry. By night, she dabbles in music, acting and writing. Her passions include faith, social justice, pan-Africanism, social justice, and mental health advocacy.

Olorunfemi Ifepade Fagunwa (she/her) is a British-Nigerian writer-director whose work focuses on the blessings and burdens of culture, domestic relationships, and how love is performed in private. In 2018, she completed the year-long Novel Studio with City University and won the Novel Studio Competition for her short story 'The Long Goodbye'. She has also written plays that have been performed at the Hampstead Theatre and Theatre Royal Stratford East and is an alumni of the Royal Court Writers Programme. When she is not writing, Olorunfemi can be found trying to live her best life away from a computer, which often involves swimming and wine but not at the same time.

Patricia Hope (she/her) is a mother of two children and was born and raised in Buckinghamshire. Her parents came to England as British Subjects from the island of St Vincent in 1959.

Raman Mundair (she/her and they/them) is an Indian-born director, award-winning author, artist, activist, filmmaker, and playwright based in Shetland and Glasgow. She is not neurotypical and identifies as disabled, Queer and a British Asian intersectional feminist. Her work includes: *Lovers, Liars, Conjurers and Thieves,* *A Choreographer's Cartography, The Algebra of Freedom* (a play), and *Incoming: Some Shetland Voices.* She is part of BBC Writersroom's Scottish Drama Writers Programme 2021 initiative and has been commissioned to develop an original drama with Synchronicity Films. You can connect with Raman at rmundair.wixsite.com/website, Twitter: @MundairRaman, Instagram: @ramanmundair + @rmundair

Raza Griffiths (he/him) is a lived experience social justice campaigner and lecturer, creating momentum for greater awareness and positive change for twenty years. Most recently, he authored the Kindred Minds BAME mental health service user led manifesto, 'A Call for Social Justice' (NSUN, 2018). He also co-ordinated consultations for the Department of Health-backed 4PI Involvement Framework (NSUN, 2014), and was a Lead Writer for the draft of the Royal College of Psychiatrists' Recovery Paper, 'A Common Purpose' (2006). He has also written for publications such as *Asylum* magazine and lectures social work, occupational therapy, and clinical psychology students at Canterbury Christ Church, Kent, Essex, Greenwich and Kent Universities. In his spare time, Raza enjoys cycling, yoga, listening to music, and learning to make perfectly round chapattis.

Reba Khatun (she/her) is a forty-something mother of two. She works in a library by day, reads in the evening and dreams of stories at night. She has published a short story, poems, and artwork in various anthologies and won the 2018 FAB Prize and made the Chicken House #Open Coop in 2020. She is currently in Birmingham writing a horror story set in Bangladesh.

Rianna Walcott

See *About the Editors*.

Ruvimbo Gumbochuma (she/her) is a British-Zimbabwean writer and singer. Her works explore various themes including identity, religion and relationships. Ruvimbo's work has been commissioned by Apples & Snakes and Beatfreaks, published by Team Angelica, Arts Council, and Verve Poetry Press. She has also facilitated poetry workshops for literary festivals such as SPINE and National Poetry Day. Ruvimbo's music has been supported by BBC Radio 1, BBC Radio 1Xtra, BBC Radio Introducing London, Reprezent Radio, Complex UK, and TRENCH, to name a few. She was also selected to join the iluvlive Artist Development programme in July 2020.

Sarah Atayero (she/her) is a British Nigerian trainee clinical psychologist at Royal Holloway, University of London and a director of the BiPP Network. Sarah's experience of working within NHS mental health services highlighted multiple challenges intersecting with her identity as a Black British woman. Consequently, Sarah's clinical practice, research, and writing are centred on exploring how the colonial history of psychological theory contributes to racial inequalities in not only the psychology curriculum but also in mental health research and treatment.

Shuranjeet Singh (he/him) is a founder and director of Taraki, a movement working with Punjabi communities reshaping approaches to mental health. Shuranjeet founded Taraki informed by his experiences of mental health challenges and wants to work towards more effective, community-centred approaches to mental health. Alongside his work with Taraki, Shuranjeet works as a mental health research consultant, sits on several boards, and is a part-time DPhil student at Oxford University.

Skye R. Tinevimbo Chirape (she/her) is a Forensic Psychology scholar and currently a Ph.D candidate and a member of the Hub for Decolonial Feminist Psychologies in Africa at the University of Cape Town, South Africa. Her Ph.D project deals with questions of borders and migration, responding to migration issues, specifically centring on African LGBT persons seeking asylum. A local of London and Cape Town, her work also focuses on ancestral ways of knowing, collective healing, decolonising work on trauma and holding space within Black communities – specifically creating gathering circles for Black and POC Queer communities.

Sophie Bass (she/her) is a London-based illustrator of mixed British and Trinidadian heritage whose work is inspired by music, social justice, mythology, and symbolism. You can find out more at www. sophiebass.co.uk

Suchandrika Chakrabarti (she/her) is a writer and podcaster from London, and you can find out more about her work from her Twitter feed: @SuchandrikaC

Tajah Hamilton (they/them) is a Black, queer non-binary poet whose body of work fucks with the system as much as their actual racialised body does.

Dr Tarek Younis (he/him) is a Senior Lecturer in Psychology at Middlesex University. He researches and writes on Islamophobia, racism in mental health, and the securitisation of clinical settings.

Temitope Fisayo (he/him) is a medical student at King's College London and a graduate of the London School of Hygiene and Tropical Medicine. He has contributed writing to the *BMJ*, the *Journal of the Royal Society of Medicine*, and the *Financial Times*.

Theophina Gabriel (she/her) is an award-winning poet, writer, and freelance artist from Slough. Her work has been published through various platforms ranging from Sistah Zine to BBC Radio 1Xtra and she holds a BA in Philosophy and Theology from the University of Oxford. She is the Founder and Editor-in-Chief of *Onyx* Magazine (@onyxmagazineox), an award-winning independent publication dedicated to championing Black creatives.

Tobi Nicole Adebajo (they/them) is an Anti-Disciplinary artist who navigates various creative / communal spheres. Tobi's creative pieces primarily focus on communing with 'the Other' via Film, Movement, Sound, Visual, and Written formats. Their works centre the depths and nuances of a variety of themes such as: Dis/Ability, Black Sexuality, Desire, Healing, Queer Love, and Yoruba traditions.

Tosin Akinkunmi (they/them) is a Nigerian-Grenadian British digital artist from Bedfordshire. A self-taught artist, Tosin's academic background in histories of race and ethnicities informs their focus and subjects, while their love for video games and graphic novels is reflected in their love of using bright, bold colours. Their artistic character and style has captured the attention of The Tate, Superdrug, and Channel 4.

Vee (she/her) is a fantasy and science fiction screenwriter from London. In 2018 she started an outdoors mental health organisation for Black women and non-binary people. She likes binge-watching shows, cats, and complaining on Twitter.

Zeena Yasin (she/her and they/them) is a digital artist, screenwriter, and poet. She holds a master's degree in Middle Eastern Politics from SOAS. She is passionate about storytelling, representing marginalised voices, and encouraging her audience to become more aligned to their values and sense of self.

About the Editors

Dr Samara Linton (she/her) is an award-winning writer and multidisciplinary content producer, best known for co-authoring *Diane Abbott: The Authorised Biography* (2020, Biteback Publishing).

Samara was born in Jamaica and moved to London as a child. After graduating from the University of Cambridge and University College London, Samara worked as a junior doctor in east London. She started writing as a freelancer while at university, and in 2016 she was awarded 'Best New Journalist' at the Ending Violence Against Women Media Awards. Since then, Samara has written for several platforms, including the BBC, *gal-dem*, *Huff-Post UK*, *Metro*, and the Royal College of Psychiatrists, and sat on the editorial board for the *BMJ*'s award-winning *Racism in Medicine* special issue (2020).

Samara has also contributed to *Rethinking Labour's Past* (2022, Bloomsbury) and *Understanding 'Race' and Ethnicity*, second edition (2019, Bristol University Press), and co-edited the Africa All-Party Parliamentary Group report, *Lessons from Ebola Affected Communities* (2016, Polygeia).

In 2019, Samara was one of six applicants selected for the BBC Production Trainee Scheme. She currently works at the BBC Audio Science Unit as an assistant producer for several BBC World Service and Radio 4 programmes. She is also pursuing an MA in Health Humanities at University College London. More information about her work can be found at samaralinton.com. She also tweets at @samara_linton

Rianna Walcott (she/her) is not yet a doctor, but may well be at the time of publication, a fact that vexes her beyond reason because it will not be on the book cover – again. Better luck next time, she supposes.

Rianna is a final-year Ph.D candidate at King's College London, researching Black identity formation and discourse patterns in Black British digital networks, and is an English Literature graduate twice over from the University of Edinburgh. Rianna is University College London's writing lab Scholar-in-Residence for 2021–2022, and co-founder of the decolonisation project *Project Myopia*, a London Arts & Humanities Partnership (LAHP)-funded initiative and website that promotes inclusivity in academia and crowd-sourced, decolonised curriculum.[15]

Rianna is a vaguely reluctant yet prolific writer and public speaker, with bylines for various publications including *The Guardian*, the BBC, *Vice*, *Dazed*, *Metro* and the Wellcome Collection, and chapters in the edited collections *So Hormonal* (Monstrous Regiment Publishing, 2020) and *Doing Equity and Diversity for Success in Higher Education: Redressing Structural Inequalities in the Academy* (Palgrave Macmillan, 2021).

In the little time left over, Rianna moonlights as a professional jazz singer with her two bands, The Rianna Walcott Band, and Ri-Ri and the White Boys. More information about her work can be found at riannawalcott.com, and she tweets at @rianna_walcott

References

1. David Harewood, *Maybe I Don't Belong Here*, Bluebird, 2021
2. Nadiya Hussain, *Finding My Voice*, Headline, 2019
3. 'Race and Ethnic Disparities denying the existence of systemic or institutional racism in the UK' (March 2021) https://assets.publishing.service.gov.uk/government/uploads/system/uploads/attachment_data/file/974507/20210331_-_CRED_Report_-_FINAL_-_Web_Accessible.pdf
4. 'Modernising the Mental Health Act: increasing choice, reducing compulsion' (Dec 2018) https://www.gov.uk/government/publications/modernising-the-mental-health-act-final-report-from-the-independent-review
5. 'Reforming the Mental Health Act: government response' (Aug 2021) https://www.gov.uk/government/consultations/reforming-the-mental-health-act/outcome/reforming-the-mental-health-act-government-response
6. 'Serenity Integrated Mentoring (SIM) and High Intensity Network FOI Part I Response' (26 July 2021) https://www.ahsnnetwork.com/app/uploads/2021/07/Serenity-Integrated-Mentoring-and-High-Intensity-Network-FOI.pdf
7. StopSIM: Mental Illness Is Not A Crime. https://stopsim.co.uk/
8. 'Response To NHS England's Statement Dated 11/05/21 In Light Of The StopSIM Coalition's Concerns Regarding The High Intensitiy Network (HIN) And Serenity Integrated Mentoring (SIM)' (May 2021) https://stopsim.co.uk/2021/05/12/response-to-nhs-englands-statement-dated-11-05-21-in-light-of-the-stopsim-coalitions-concerns-

regarding-the-high-intensity-network-hin-and-serenity-integrated-mentoring-sim/#:~:text=We%20reiterate%20our%20call%20to,High%20Intensity%20Network%20(HIN).

9. 'Cactus Mental Health Survey Report' (2020) https://cactusglobal.com/mental-health-survey/

10. 'Narrative Experiences Online' (2017–2019) https://www.researchintorecovery.com/research/neon/

11. Ibid.

12. https://www.thestabilitynetwork.org/

13. https://www.facebook.com/thecolourofmadnessplay/

14. 'Narrative Experiences Online' (2017–2019) https://www.researchintorecovery.com/research/neon/

15. www.projectmyopia.com

Index

Note: page numbers in **bold** refer to illustrations.

benefits 112
benzodiazepines 115
Bible
   Corinthians 84
   Leviticus 251
   Psalms 253, 256, 257
bipolar disorder 52, 57, 111–12
bisexuality 130–5, 140
Black African patients 208
Black agency staff 199
Black, Asian and minority ethnic
   (BAME) 3, 4, 42
   children 107
   see also Black, minority ethnic
Black Caribbean patients 208
Black children 131
Black communities 43
Black history 45
Black, minority ethnic (BME) 174,
   199, 200
Black narratives 45
Black people 180, 209
   and Christianity 253
   discrimination against 193
   increased likelihood of mental
     health sectioning 252–3
   marginalisation 191
   patients 192–3, 196, 206, 208–9
   predisposition to mental health
     problems 200
   women 109, 114–16
Blackness 40, 181
blood donation 228–9
Blue Smile 107
body
   Black 181
   marginalised 180
   objectification 166
brain chemistry 57
brain fog 255

Brazil 99
breakdowns 56, 68, 230–5
breathing techniques 17, 23
British Caribbeans 114–15
brothers 76–8
bulimia nervosa 79–83
bullying 133, 135–6
busy lives, glamorisation 171

Camden 91, 96
cancer 93
cannabis 42
capitalism 163
   see also anti-capitalism
'Captive Maternals' 232, 233
carers, young 98
caretaking 232
certainty 219
   see also uncertainty
Charhdi Kala 56
Chauhan, Hima, *Magaj* **150**, 166–7
Chidune, Avila Diana, *The History
   of Yellow* **154**
childhood abuse 285
   sexual 121, 122, 140
children 107, 130–43
   care-experienced 98
   and depression 135
Christianity 253–4, 257
circle imagery 173–4
Clash, The 177
class 126
   inequality 106–7
clozapine 94–5
colonialism 127
community
   belonging 220–1
   community-based solutions
     214–15
   counselling initiatives 43

seasonal affective disorder (S.A.D.) 258–9

sectioning 98, 195, 198, 208, 252–3

see also Mental Health Act

sedatives 114–15

selective serotonin reuptake inhibitors (SSRIs) 262–3

see also sertraline

self, Black 181

self-care 127

self-compassion 51–2, 126

self-harm 41, 42, 82, 110–11, 114, 206–7, 232, 277

self-hatred 41

self-love 261–2

self-medicating 42, 82

self-worth 40, 222

Serenity Integrated Mentoring (SIM) scheme 5

sertraline 129, 261–3

sex 278

Sex Pistols, The 177

sexual abuse 121, 122, 140

sexual assault 110, 166, 231–5

sexual orientation 130–5

shame 52, 54, 123, 219–20

Sikhi 56–8, 211

slavery 212–13

sleeping pills 230

smoking 60–1, 64–5

'snowflakes' 13, 52

social connection 173–4, 176, 302

social inequality 211

social isolation 43

self-imposed 11

see also loneliness

social media 5

Sohanpal, David, *Moon* 155

Soho Radio 91–2

solicitors 226

somatic work 44

South Asian women 166, 167

spaces 44–5

Spilfest Eating Disorders Unit 72–8

SSRIs *see* selective serotonin reuptake inhibitors

Stability Network 101

'stateless persons' 222

status quo, inability to fit 44

STEM *see* Science, Technology, Engineering and Mathematics

stereotypes
cultural 166
dependency 166
racist 211
reductionist 211

stigma
and antidepressants 261, 263
and mental illness 55
and suicide 53–8

Stirling, Tabatha 2–3
Stirling Publishing Limited 2–3

StopSIM Coalition 5

stress
chronic 124
post-traumatic 126, 198

students 180–2, 231–5

substance abuse 42, 57
see also alcohol consumption

suffering 257

suicidal ideation 111, 114, 232, 235, 255, 257

suicide
attempted 164–5, 195, 198, 239–44
stigma of 53–8

superimposition 177–8

support systems 256–7

support workers 206–9

Permissions Acknowledgements